# Molecular Mechanisms of the Immune Response

# CANCER SURVEYS

## Advances and Prospects in Clinical, Epidemiological and Laboratory Oncology



Published for the

**Imperial Cancer** Research Fund

# Molecular Mechanisms of the Immune Response

Guest Editors

W F Bodmer

M J Owen

COLD SPRING HARBOR LABORATORY PRESS 1995

**CANCER SURVEYS**
*Molecular Mechanisms of the Immune Response*
Volume 22


Published by Cold Spring Harbor Laboratory Press
Printed in the United States of America
ISBN 0-87969-442-4
ISSN 0261-2429

*Cover and book design by Leon Bolognese & Associates, Inc.*



All Cold Spring Harbor Laboratory Press publications may be ordered directly from Cold Spring Harbor Laboratory Press, 10 Skyline Drive, Plainview, New York 11803-9729. Phone: Continental US & Canada 1-800-843-4388; all other locations (516) 349-1930. FAX: (516) 349-1946.

# Contents

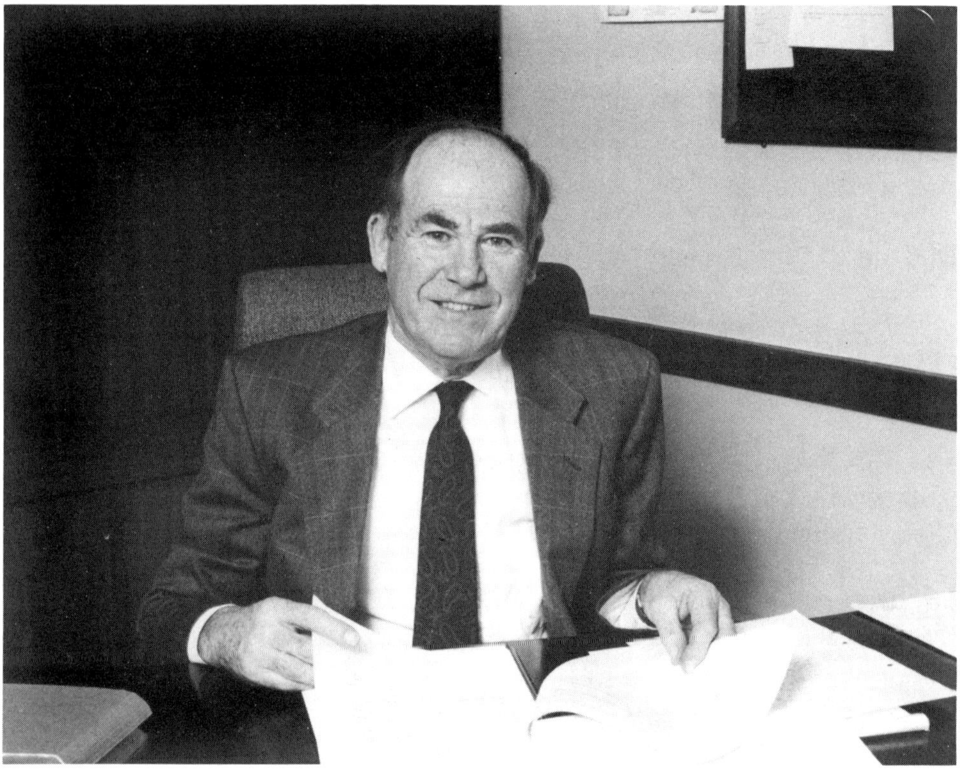

*This volume of Cancer Surveys is dedicated to Michael Crumpton, Ph.D., CBE., FRS, on the occasion of his retirement as Director of Research (Laboratories) at the Imperial Cancer Research Fund, after many years of outstanding and dedicated service.*

# Introduction

**W F BODMER • M J OWEN**
*Imperial Cancer Research Fund, 44 Lincoln's Inn Fields, London WC2A 3PX*

This volume of *Cancer Surveys* honours Dr Mike Crumpton on the occasion of his retirement as Director of Research (Laboratories) at the Imperial Cancer Research Fund. It is based on a scientific symposium held at the Royal Society on 11 October 1993. The title of the symposium, "The Lymphocyte Cell Surface", reflected Mike's major area of interest for much of his scientific life, and one to which he has made so many contributions.

As an undergraduate at the end of the war, Mike read chemistry at Southampton University (then a college of London University) on a scholarship. At that time, most school-leavers were required to undertake a period of National Service, most university places being reserved for forces' educational training, although an exception was made for students who attained university scholarships. During this time, Mike developed an interest in biochemistry, despite the disapproval of the head of school, Professor NK Adam, who was an eminent surface chemist. Fortunately, Mike was introduced to the Lister Institute by Margary Ish-Campbell and undertook a PhD with Walter Morgan in carbohydrate chemistry, working on the chemical basis of blood group ABO specificity.

After completing his PhD studies, Mike could no longer evade National Service and was seconded first to the David Bruce laboratories on Salisbury Plain. There, Mike received a training in microbiology, working with James Howard. He was then posted to DAL Davies' laboratory at the Microbiological Research Establishment at Porton, working on immune responses to plague.

At the end of his period of National Service, Mike stayed on briefly as a member of the scientific civil service before undertaking a postdoctoral period in the USA. Even at that formative stage of his career, Mike realized the potential power of a rigorous quantitative biochemical approach to immunology and consequently undertook a postdoctoral period in the laboratory of one of the world's leading protein chemists, Christian Anfinsen. There, Mike worked with Dreyer and Streisinger, who had initiated studies on phage lysozyme mutants in experiments designed to establish the co-linearity of the genetic code. Although these experiments met with mixed success, they gave him a grounding in protein chemistry that was to become such a feature of his scientific work.

After his sojourn at the National Institutes of Health, Mike returned to the UK, joining Professor Rodney Porter's department at St Mary's Hospital

*Cancer Surveys* Volume 22: *Molecular Mechanisms of the Immune Response*

Medical School. Rod Porter exerted a major influence over Mike's career, and indeed over British immunology, until his tragic and untimely death in 1985. There, Mike undertook a study designed to elucidate the molecular basis of antigenicity. He chose to dissect the rabbit antibody response to sperm whale myoglobin, a small globular protein that was in plentiful supply and the X ray structure of which had been determined to 2.2 Å resolution by Kendrew's group in Cambridge. In a meticulous series of experiments, Mike localized some of the major antigenic regions of myoglobin and, in a short paper to the *Journal of Molecular Biology,* proposed the concept that antigenic peptides could adopt an equilibrium of conformations and that an antibody binding site could select a particular conformation, thus displacing the equilibrium. This concept of protein "breathing" was proposed independently by Anfinsen in his Nobel prize winning studies on the denaturation and refolding of RNase S.

By now firmly established as a biochemical immunologist, Mike Crumpton's next move was to the division of biochemistry at the National Institute for Medical Research at Mill Hill. At that time, NIMR was a Mecca for immunological research, with such luminaries as Av Mitchison, John Humphrey and Ite Askonas, and also for protein chemistry. It was thus a natural choice. His time at NIMR was associated with two major areas of research. He initiated an enduring interest in T cell activation, and, together with Michael Green, was first to show using the A23187 calcium ionophore that a rise in intracellular [$Ca^{2+}$] was sufficient to initiate the complex process of T cell activation. He also began his studies on the purification of lymphocyte plasma membranes which would form the basis of his work on the characterization of the human class I and class II histocompatibility antigens. These latter studies were undertaken as a long collaboration with one of us (WFB) that was a major influence on the remainder of Mike's scientific career. The availability of highly purified plasma membrane from large quantities of B lymphoblastoid cells and the demonstration that the lectin purified from lentils could be used to purify detergent solubilized membrane glycoproteins were key developments in the successful purification of the HLA-A, -B, -C and -DR antigens.

During Mike Crumpton's tenure at NIMR, progress in our understanding of the major histocompatibility complex (MHC) was rapid. The overall structures of class I and class II antigens had been elucidated and the functions of these molecules as guidance systems for T cells had been firmly established. Indeed, the pioneering experiment by Zinkernagel and Doherty that defined MHC restriction had been carried out at the John Curtin School of Medicine in Australia when Mike was on sabbatical leave there in 1973. The elegant experiments of the Crumpton/Bodmer laboratories on the purification of HLA-A, -B, -C and -DR antigens in amounts sufficient for biochemical analysis were carried out with the firm conviction that structural knowledge of a protein would illuminate its function. How right this conviction was, as so dramatically illustrated by the subsequent work, over a decade later, by Wiley's group on the three dimensional structures of class I and class II antigens.

Perhaps Mike's major regret in his scientific life was that he chose not to follow up the protein chemistry with detailed structural analysis of histocompatibility antigens. This decision was in part due to the philosophy that a scientist should eschew "obvious" experiments and constantly blaze new conceptual trails, leaving others to follow up. The impact of our knowledge of the three dimensional structures of histocompatibility antigens on immunology surely shows how simplistic this philosophy can sometimes be.

Mike's next move was to the Imperial Cancer Research Fund as Deputy Director of Research in 1979. With WFB as Director of Research, the Oxford/NIMR collaboration was united. However, active, scientific collaboration between the two laboratories was less than when they were situated in different cities. A number of reasons contributed to this: recombinant DNA technology had begun to make an impact on MHC genetics, and Mike had developed an interest in the structure and function of surface molecules, such as the CD2 and CD3 antigens involved in T cell activation. Mike also continued studies on the intracellular events associated with T cell activation, concentrating on phosphorylation events and on a family of calcium binding proteins known as the annexins. He continued to make major contributions in these areas despite shouldering an increasingly large burden of administrative responsibility both at the ICRF and in a variety of outside contexts.

There are a number of hallmarks of excellence in a scientific career. A scientist is often judged by the subsequent careers of people who have trained in his or her laboratory. There are a variety of successful scientists around the world who have passed through Mike's lab or who have been influenced by him in collaborative studies. Perhaps the most satisfying hallmark is to be able to have made fundamental contributions to one's field and to see these contributions form a platform for much of the subsequent work in the field. The articles that comprise this volume of *Cancer Surveys* provide ample evidence of the impact of Mike Crumpton's research and underscore the power of molecular approaches to the study of complex biological systems such as the immune response.

# Evolution and Function of the HLA Region

**WALTER F BODMER**
*Imperial Cancer Research Fund, Lincoln's Inn Fields, London WC2A 3PX*



## INTRODUCTION

The HLA, H2 and other major histocompatibility systems were discovered, by analogy with the human red cell bloodgroups, in the search for polymorphic antigens to match for transplantation. Subsequently, they have been shown to have a key functional role in immune response, and their membership of the immunoglobulin supergene family suggested the name "histoglobulins" (Bodmer, 1989).

The first experimental clue to a relationship between the HLA gene products and immunoglobulins came from the fact that the HLA class I associated molecule $\beta_2$ microglobulin had a sequence that predicted an immunoglobulin related structure. Subsequently, partial aminoacid sequence analysis of HLA class I gene products, and complete sequences derived from the cloned genes, showed clearly that the membrane proximal domains of HLA class I and class II products were members of the immunoglobulin supergene family. The N-terminal domains, however, did not fit this structure, and it was not until the determination of the HLA-A2 structure by Bjorkman *et al* (1987) that the significance of this domain as a peptide clamp became clear. Thus, the function of the HLA molecules was shown to be to hold peptides derived from endogenous or exogenous proteins by specific proteolytic degradation in a position such that they could be specifically recognized by the T cell receptor. The structural data furthermore confirmed the immunoglobulin homology of the membrane proximal domain, and similar data have now been obtained from Wiley and Strominger and their colleagues for the HLA class II structure (Brown *et al,* 1993).

*Cancer Surveys* Volume 22: *Molecular Mechanisms of the Immune Response*

The immunoglobulin homology supported speculative suggestions that the evolutionary precursor of the HLA region products may have a role in cellular recognition and cell-cell interaction during differentiation and development (Bodmer, 1972; Gally and Edelman, 1972). This idea is now further supported by the discovery by Edelman and others of a variety of cellular adhesion molecules, which are indeed also members of the immunoglobulin supergene family (Edelman, 1992).

## EVOLUTION OF THE HLA REGION

The key event during the very early evolution of the HLA system genes must have been the fusion of the gene for an immunoglobulin domain, possibly derived from a cellular adhesion molecular function, with a gene for a peptide binding domain, perhaps derived from a gene for a heat shock protein or one of its ancestors (Fig. 1) (Bodmer, 1992). This event, which must have taken place at least 5–7 hundred million years ago in early Cambrian or even pre-Cambrian organisms, was followed by a series of duplications and divergence, leading eventually to the present set of genes. The early stages of this process were at a time when there appears to have been a very rapid evolution of these and related functional genes, perhaps shortly after the major initial evolutionary development of multicellular eukaryotic organisms. The first HLA molecule was probably a homodimer of a fused immunoglobulin and peptide binding domain analogous to the HLA class II molecules. Class I molecules could then have arisen in two different ways, either by duplication of the N-terminal peptide binding domain of such an initial primitive histoglobulin molecule or by an independent fusion event between the genes for an immunoglobulin domain and an already duplicated peptide binding domain. In either case, the complete class I molecule needs an additional free immunoglobulin domain, now represented by $\beta_2$ microglobulin.

Duplication and divergence of the original histoglobulin gene formed by an immunoglobulin and peptide binding domain fusion will have given rise to the original class II $\alpha/\beta$ heterodimer. Further divergence of the separate class II A and B genes, followed by duplication, then led to the *DPB, DQB, DRB, DPA, DQA* and *DRA* sets of genes. An analogous series of steps following the formation of the initial gene for the class I precursor will have given rise to the class I genes now seen in the HLA region.

Periods of expansion and contraction of closely related sets of genes, such as *DRB* and *DPA* and *DPB,* during mammalian evolution and no doubt also earlier have resulted in differences in the representation of these various genes in different species including, in particular, humans, and mice (for earlier discussion of these evolutionary ideas, see Travers *et al,* 1984; Bodmer *et al,* 1986; Bodmer, 1992).

The recently described *DMA* and *DMB* genes (Kelly and Trowsdale, 1994) are intriguing in that they have an overall class II like structure but have se-

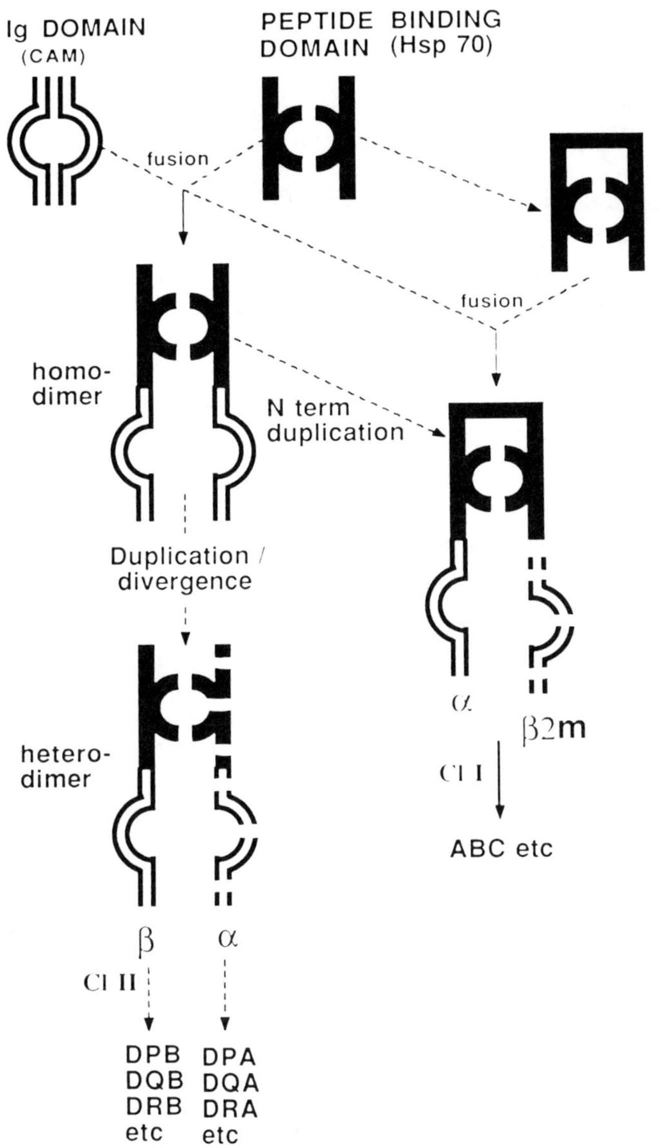


**Fig. 1.** Scheme for early evolution of the HLA system

quences that show no greater homology with class II than with class I. This suggests a very early separation between this *DM* pair and the others, after the initial evolution of class II A and B genes. These genes are much less polymorphic than the classical HLA class II genes, other than *DRA,* and may have some rather specific function connected with class II based recognition that perhaps does not require interaction with a very wide range of peptides. Kasahara *et al* (1992) have isolated a typical mammalian like class II α chain from a nurse shark (*Ginglymostoma cirratum*), suggesting that the basic divergence of histoglobulins into class I and class II as we now know them most probably predated the appearance of cartilaginous fishes. They find that

HLA *DMA* has the strongest sequence homology with their shark class II *A* gene.

## The HLA Region Map: An Evolutionary Interpretation

More and more genes are being found in the HLA region, especially between the class I and class II clusters (see Campbell and Trowsdale, 1993). The region as a whole consists of some 3.5 million base pairs, extending from somewhere between the collagen gene for type IIAII and *DPB2* to the end of the class I region, so far defined by HLA-F. This size estimate, now made precise by genomic analysis using yeast artificial chromosomes, has remained remarkably stable over a period of nearly 25 years. The overall genomic organization in humans and mice is extraordinarily similar, but there is polymorphism in the HLA region for the number of genes and their arrangement around *DRB2* and the C4 complement gene cluster.

There are three major categories of genes in the HLA region:

(a) The HLA class I genes, including several in addition to those for A, B and C, the class II genes, including *DMA, DMB* and *DNA*, and various related pseudogenes.
(b) Other genes with immune related functions. The first to be found were the complement genes for C4, C2 and Bf and then *TNFA* and *TNFB* in the region between the class I and class II clusters. More recently, and strikingly, there has been the discovery through genomic analysis of the class II region of the transporter and proteasome component genes *TAP1* and *TAP2* and *LMP2* and *LMP7*. The discovery of a small cluster of *Hsp70* genes (*HSPA*) in the middle of the HLA region is intriguing, although their apparent specificity for the testis makes a role for them in immune response unlikely. The class II equivalents of the transporters also remain to be clearly identified.
(c) Many other genes with functions unrelated to the immune system. These include, for example, the 21-hydroxylase genes, a gene for a tenascin related molecule, the gene for valyl-t-RNA synthetase and a number of other genes whose function has yet to be determined.

The strong human-mouse homology of the map implies that the overall arrangement is common, at least to mammals, apart from minor perturbations due to local expansion and contraction of duplicated genes. It seems possible that this overall organization reflects the collection of genes that surrounded the primitive precursor of the histoglobulin genes formed from the immunoglobulin and peptide binding domain fusion. The various duplications followed by divergence are then presumed to have occurred within and around this collection of genes, leading to the present organization. Duplicates could easily have been spread locally by, for example, association with an intrachromosomal inversion giving rise to the gap between the class I and the class II genes. It is notable that there are relatively few, if any, non-immune function genes within the class II region. There is also a suggestion of a further major rearrangement which separated HLA-A and the associated cluster of class I genes from HLA-B and C. It remains to be seen whether the gap between A and B,C will contain as divergent a set of genes with respect to function as does the gap between B,C and the class II region.

There is no reason why the duplicate genes that led to the evolution of the HLA class I and class II genes should have been separated during evolution. The separation would have required specific selection, either for a translocation or for a transposed gene. The duplicate genes have presumably "co-adapted" following their divergence, and favourable combinations have no doubt been held together from time to time by interactive selection, resulting in linkage disequilibrium.

It seems likely, as suggested originally for the complement genes, that some of the immune function genes that are not HLA class I or class II genes could have been "brought in" to the HLA region by selection. Thus, selection favouring a particular combination of one of the "brought in" genes, say a transporter, and a particular pre-existing HLA region gene would favour, through linkage disequilibrium, a transposition that brought the two together. Once this combination had swept through a population, the reorganization would be established and there would need to be no residual selective interaction between the two genes to maintain the new arrangement.

There remain at least two major puzzles. Where are the human equivalents of the mouse *TL* and *QA* genes, which appear to be peptide receptors, although perhaps of more limited specificity (Rotzschke *et al,* 1993) and perhaps specialized to recognizing $\delta/\gamma$ T cells, as proposed by Tonegawa and colleagues (Wu *et al,* 1991)? If these molecules have a special role in recognizing a more specific restricted class of determinants, or do so in selected tissues, then where is the equivalent human function? It is not clear whether the atypical class I genes such as those for HLA E, F and G necessarily fulfil this role.

The second puzzle relates to the origin of the *CD1* genes and their functions. These are clearly class I like genes associated with $\beta_2$ microglobulin but which map outside the HLA region (Calabi and Milstein, 1986). Do these also have a function that is tissue specific or more restricted than the other HLA class I genes? And what is their origin? Were they an early transposition of class I region genes to another part of the genome, or were the original class I genes transposed into what we now call the HLA region during a very early stage in its evolution?

## HLA CLASS II FUNCTION AND POLYMORPHISM

The basic function of class II molecules is to present peptides, derived from exogenous proteins, to T cell receptors on CD4 positive cells. The class II molecules are expressed constitutively at a high level on specialized antigen presenting cells, especially dendritic cells, as well as on B lymphocytes, where their function is presumably to present peptides from proteins recognized by the specific antibody on the surface of the B lymphocyte to promote T-B interaction for the stimulation of antibody production. It is clear now that class II molecules are more promiscuous than class I molecules with respect to the range of peptides that can be bound by any particular allelic combination (Brown *et al,* 1993). From a functional point of view, it would appear likely that class II/T cell receptor interactions were associated with the evolution of the antibody production system, and that is likely to have followed the more primitive direct T cell cytotoxic recognition system. This would not be consistent with an evolution of class I from class II molecules but leaves open the question of whether the homodimer postulated in Fig. 1 was in fact the common precursor of both class I and class II molecules.

The fact that most of the DNA sequence differences between polymorphic alleles, whether of class II or class I products, give rise to aminoacid substitutions and occur in restricted positions that are now seen to correspond to the peptide binding regions is strong evidence for the role of selection in generating these polymorphisms (Bodmer *et al,* 1986). This follows from a principle first clearly enunciated by Luca Cavalli-Sforza that, when there is differential variation, this cannot be explained by population structure effects, namely the combination of mutation and random drift (Cavalli-Sforza and Bodmer, 1972). This is because the effects of population structure will apply equally to all regions of a gene, whatever their functional significance, and so the sort of differential variation associated with the peptide binding region cannot be explained by the combination of mutation and random drift.

It is striking that for the DR molecules, essentially only the DR β chain varies, whereas for DQ and DP, both α and β chains vary. There is no doubt that there must be some functional differentiation between these three sets of molecules, although whether it is simply that DR is involved in help and DQ in suppression is, I believe, unlikely. It seems more probable that the different sets of molecules provide different spectra of efficiency of antigen recognition. The diversification of both class II and class I molecules may thus represent a fine tuning of the immune system, providing an increase in the efficiency with which a broad spectrum of peptides can be handled. There may also be an element of tissue specificity, since it seems likely that the induction of class II expression by, for example, γ interferon in a wide variety of tissues provides a mechanism whereby a cell from any tissue may at first act as an antigen presenting cell. The class II *DP* genes may be switched on earlier by γ interferon in at least some cell types, such as epithelial cells, than are the other class II genes (Balkwill *et al,* 1987). Perhaps, therefore, *DP* genes have a specific role in antigen presentation to CD4 T helper cells when they are expressed on "non-professional" antigen presenting cells, such as epithelial cells.

It is important to distinguish the origin of a polymorphic variant, by mutation, recombination or gene conversion, from its propagation into a population, namely its increase in frequency. As already pointed out, mutation and random drift are in general most unlikely to be the forces that have driven HLA region allelic variants to relatively high frequencies. Mutation is simply not a significant driving force in comparison with selection.

Since the original description by McDevitt and Benacceraf of immune response differences associated with the mouse H2 polymorphism more than 25 years ago, it has been obvious that immune response variation with respect to pathogens, whether bacteria, viruses, protozoan parasites or fungi, is likely to be the major basis for the effect of natural selection on HLA polymorphism. Some form of frequency dependent or fluctuating selection, in which different alleles were favoured at different times, may be the major mechanism maintaining the high level of HLA polymorphism (Bodmer, 1972). Such a mechanism gives heterozygote advantage over time but does not require any particular heterozygote at any given time to be at an advantage, as has been argued by Hughes and Nei (1989). Their suggestion that such specific heterozygote advantage arises because of a doubling of the opportunity for different sorts of immune responses does not seem plausible since, as Muller first suggested, if this was a requirement then it would be satisfied much better by increasing the number of duplicate genes.

The patterns of variation between alleles suggest that it may be combinations of epitopes that are selected for and that new combinations can be formed from old by recombination, as is particularly clear for the *DP* variations. This is an old idea that goes back to Fisher's interpretation of the rhesus blood groups and to the earliest interpretations of the HLA system in the mid 1960s. If different epitope combinations are present in a population at low frequencies, maintained by recurrent mutation or perhaps more likely by recombination and conversion, then, when the selective situation requires it, a new combination may quickly increase in frequency to cope with a new immune challenge. Thus, fluctuating selection can readily be responded to by extensive polymorphism but not simply by an increase in the number of genes. Heterozygote advantage per se does not allow this flexibility of response. The long persistence of alleles across species seems most likely to reflect the existence of tried and trusted epitopes for peptide binding and their combinations.

Within a closely linked cluster of genes, such as in the HLA region, if there is one variant on a particular haplotype that is selected for, then linkage disequilibrium will ensure that the haplotype as a whole will tend to increase in frequency by the phenomenon called "hitch-hiking" by Maynard-Smith, first analysed by Bodmer and Parsons (1962). The essential point is that, during a relatively rapid increase in frequency, there is not enough time for recombination to disrupt the association between the selected allele and other alleles on the haplotype initially associated with the selected allele. Thus, in my view, the so called extended haplotypes are simply a reflection of relatively rapid selection for one particular allele within those haplotypes in the relevant populations. Of course, from time to time, there may well be co-ordinated selection for alleles at two or more different loci with immune functions on the same haplotype, leading to the types of selective interaction that would accentuate the observation of an apparently extended haplotype.

## HLA CLASS I FUNCTION

The basic function of class I molecules is to present peptides derived from the processing of endogenous proteins to the T cell receptor on cytotoxic CD8 T cells (Townsend and Bodmer, 1989). This process ensures that no virus can hide within a cell, because it should always leave a signature of processed peptides derived from its expressed genes held on the surface by HLA class I products ready to be recognized by specific cytotoxic T cells. The power of this recognition system is no doubt why viruses have evolved a wide variety of mechanisms to escape from the immune response. These include a range of devices for downregulating the expression of surface HLA class I molecules.

HLA class I molecules appear to be less promiscuous with respect to the variety of peptides they can bind than are class II molecules. A priori this would appear to be a disadvantage, since it apparently limits the potential range of immune responses. This is no doubt why the Epstein-Barr virus, when it has transformed a cell and requires only the expression of EBNA I to maintain the transformed state, cannot be recognized by the immune system. It appears that EBNA I may have evolved in such a way that it does not give rise to any processed peptides that can be recognized. It has, in other words, evolved to be effectively a universally "tolerant" protein. On the other hand, if the HLA class I molecules were too promiscuous with respect to their binding specificity, then perhaps tolerance would be broken too easily, leading rather readily to autocytotoxicity. It seems quite plausible that breaking tolerance in this way with respect to class I and cytotoxic T cell determinants could be much more damaging than breaking tolerance by the production of autoantibodies, which are after all quite common and apparently mostly without pathogenic effects in older people. So the comparatively restricted range of peptides recognized by class I molecules may reflect a balance between limiting damaging autoimmunity and nevertheless providing an adequate range of responses to peptide from processed foreign proteins.

Van Rood and his colleagues (Claas *et al,* 1988) have described the phenomenon of tolerance, with respect to antibody production, to non-inherited maternal HLA antigens. This may be correlated with breastfeeding and the induction of tolerance by maternal lymphocytes present in the milk. This fits with the observation (Campbell *et al,* 1984) that mother to child kidney transplants do significantly better if the child has been breastfed. It has often been pointed out that early acquired immunity from breastfeeding may be an important protection mechanism before the full development of an infant's immune system. This has, however, mostly been thought of in terms of passively-transmitted antibodies. It seems, however, most likely that the same will occur with respect to passively transmitted T cells. It is, after all, common practice not to vaccinate before about 3 months of age because it requires roughly that period of time before an infant has built up a sufficient variety of immune responses to cope on its own. Perhaps evolution has ensured that during this early period the infant is tolerant to the cells acquired from the mother through the milk, and thus acquires the mother's T and B cell immunity during this critical early stage of its life. This, then, could readily account for tolerance to the non-inherited maternal antigens associated with extended survival of maternal T cells acquired during the earliest stages of breastfeeding. There is an important general corollary that follows if this idea is correct. This is that an individual's immune system may be significantly influenced at an early stage by maternally acquired immune T lymphocytes through breastfeeding and, particularly, by the absence of breastfeeding. It might therefore be worth exploring the association between breastfeeding and immune related disorders such as allergy, asthma and autoimmune diseases such as insulin dependent juvenile onset diabetes and rheumatoid arthritis.

## HLA EXPRESSION, FETAL-MATERNAL IMMUNITY AND TUMOUR IMMUNITY

It has been known for some time that the majority of trophoblasts do not express HLA-A, B and C molecules. This still seems by far the most likely mechanism by which the fetus survives as an allograft, since this ensures that the tissue in closest contact with the maternal circulation can neither be recognized as different by cytotoxic T cells nor stimulate them to respond (Barnstable and Bodmer, 1978). It is interesting in this context that McMichael and colleagues (Ellis *et al,* 1990) have shown that HLA-G is expressed on at least some trophoblasts but is essentially non-polymorphic. This, together with a ready induction of HLA A,B,C expression following viral challenge, may ensure that ultimately the fetus and so the mother may be protected from infection. However, this may sometimes be at the cost of losing an embryo, and perhaps this explains some of the damage associated with certain viral infections during early pregnancy.

The observation of a lack of surface HLA A,B,C expression on the Burkitt's lymphoma derived cell line, Daudi, associated with the idea of the role of lack of HLA A,B,C expression in protecting a cell against immune T cell attack led to the suggestion that tumour escape from T cell attack may also involve selection for reduced or absent HLA A,B,C expression (Barnstable and Bodmer, 1978; Brodsky *et al,* 1979). Many subsequent studies have confirmed the relatively common loss either of overall HLA A,B,C expression or of expression of individual alleles. This, together with the knowledge that a T cell can recognize intracellular determinants, so making any oncogene change, and indeed tumour suppressor gene mutation, a potential target for the immune system, has revolutionized our views on tumour immunity and the potential for tumour immunotherapy and even vaccination (for review, see eg Bodmer *et al,* 1993).

Recently, a study of $\beta_2$ microglobulin gene mutations in established colorectal carcinoma cell lines and fresh tumours has revealed a significant frequency of such mutations reflecting direct selection for reduced HLA class I expression or complete loss of expression. Thus, the colorectal carcinoma derived cell line Lovo, which was the first human carcinoma to be shown to lack completely surface HLA A,B,C expression, is a homo- or hemizygous $\beta_2$ microglobulin mutation. This arose from a mutation in the $\beta_2$ microglobulin leader sequence that gives rise to a non-functional protein, followed most probably by non-disjunction leading to loss of the wild type $\beta_2$ microglobulin gene (Bicknell *et al,* 1994).

Out of a total of eight $\beta_2$ microglobulin mutations observed in a screen of 37 colorectal carcinoma derived cell lines and 22 fresh tumours, two of the cell lines were heterozygous for a $\beta_2$ microglobulin mutation and so retained HLA A,B,C and $\beta_2$ microglobulin surface expression, but at a reduced level. This is consistent with the fact that each genetic step during tumour progression must be selected for. This implies that if two mutational steps are needed to eliminate HLA A,B,C expression, for example, recessive mutations knocking out the function of both copies of the $\beta_2$ microglobulin gene as in the Daudi and Lovo cell lines, then the first mutation must on its own confer a selective advantage. Since the only known function of $\beta_2$ microglobulin is as a component of HLA class I and related molecules and their involvement in the immune response, the only basis for the selection of $\beta_2$ microglobulin mutations must be escape from T cell immune response.

The frequency with which significant changes in HLA expression, including individual HLA class I allele loss, has been observed, at least in colorectal carcinomas, suggests that T cell responses to tumours may be more common than was, at least until recently, supposed to be the case. In most cases, it appears that this response may be too weak, or occur too late, to have a significant effect on prognosis. Nevertheless, the existence of such responses does provide hope that more aggressive responses may be induced at relatively early stages of tumour progression as a basis for tumour immunotherapy. It may also be possible to induce immunity to oncogene mutations, such as RAS, TP53 or truncated APC gene products, as a basis for genuine vaccination against cancers not associated with viruses. This is just one application that flows from our enormous increase in understanding of the basic functions of the genes of the HLA region and, more generally, of the mechanisms of T and B cell immunity.

## Acknowledgements

I am very happy to acknowledge many productive years of collaboration with Mike Crumpton, which educated me in the biochemistry of surface proteins and have greatly influenced my thoughts on the HLA system, its function and evolution.

## References

Balkwill FR, Proietti E, Bodmer J, Hart I and Ramani P (1987) Mechanisms of antitumour actions of interferons on human tumour xenografts and in mouse metastases models. *European Journal of Cancer* **23** 101–106

Barnstable CJ and Bodmer WF (1978) Immunology and the fetus. *Lancet* **i** 326

Bicknell DC, Rowan A and Bodmer WF (1994) Beta2 microglobulin gene mutations: a study of established colorectal cell lines and fresh tumors. *Proceedings of the National Academy of Sciences of the USA* **91** 4751–4755

Bjorkman PJ, Saper MA, Samraoui B, Bennett WS, Strominger JL and Wiley DC (1987) Structure of the human classI histocompatibility antigen HLA-A2. *Nature* **329** 506–512

Bodmer WF (1972) Evolutionary significance of the HL-A system. *Nature* **237** 139–145

Bodmer WF (1989) HLA 1987 immunology of HLA, In: Dupont B (ed). *Immunogenetics and Histocompatibility,* vol 2, pp 1–9, Springer, New York

Bodmer WF (1992) HLA 1991 *Proceedings of the Eleventh International Histocompatibility Workshop and Conference* **1** 7–16

Bodmer WF and Parsons PA (1962) Linkage and recombinationin evolution. *Advances in Genetics* **11** 1–100

Bodmer WF, Trowsdale J, Young J and Bodmer J (1986) Gene clusters and the evolution of the major histocompatibility system. *Philosophical Transactions of the Royal Society of London, Series B* **312** 303–315

Bodmer WF, Browning MF, Krausa P, Rowan A, Bicknell DC and Bodmer JGB (1993) Tumour escape from immune response by variation in HLA expressions and other mechanisms. *Annals of the New York Academy of Sciences* **690** 42–49

Brodsky FM, Parham P, Barnstable CJ, Crumpton MJ and Bodmer WF (1979) Monoclonal antibodies for analysis ofthe HLA system. *Immunological Reviews* **47** 3–61

Brown JH, Jardetzky TS, Gorga JC *et al* (1993) Three-dimensional structure of the human class II histocompatibility antigen HLA-DR1. *Nature* **364** 33–39

Calabi F and Milstein C (1986) A novel family of human major histocompatibility complex-related genes not mapping to chromosome. *Nature* **323** 540–543

Campbell DA Jr, Lorber MI, Sweeton JC, Turcotte JG, Niederhuber JE and Beer AE (1984) Breast feeding and maternal-donor renal allografts. *Transplantation* **37** 340–344

Campbell DA and Trowsdale J (1993) Map of the human MHC. *Immunology Today* **14** 349–352

Cavalli-Sforza LL and Bodmer WF (eds) (1972) *The Genetics of Human Populations*, Freeman, San Francisco

Claas FHJ, Gijbels Y, Van der Velden-de Munck J and van Rood JJ (1988) Induction of B cell unresponsiveness to noninherited maternal HLA antigens during fetal life. *Science* **241** 1815–1817

Edelman GM (1992) Mediation and inhibition of cell-adhesion by morphoregulatory molecules. *Cold Spring Harbor Symposium of Quantitative Biology* **57** 317–325

Ellis SA, Palmer MS and McMichael AJ (1990) Human trophoblast and the choriocarcinoma cell line BeWo express a truncated HLA class I molecule. *Journal of Immunology* **144** 731–735

Gally JA and Edelman GM (1972) The genetic control of immunoglobulin synthesis. *Annual Review of Genetics* **6** 1–46

Hughes AL and Nei M (1989) Nucleotide substitution at major histocompatibility complex class II loci: evidence for overdominant selection. *Proceedings of the National Academy of Sciences of the USA* **86** 958–962

Kelly A and Trowsdale J (1994) Novel genes in the human major histocompatibility complex class-II region. *International Archives of Allergy and Immunology* **103** 11–15

Kasahara M, Vazquez M, Sato K McKinney EC and Flajnik MF (1992) Evolution of the major histocompatibility complex: isolation of class II A cDNA clones from the cartilaginous fish. *Proceedings of the National Academy of Sciences of the USA* **896** 688–6692

Rotzschke O, Falk K, Stevanovic S *et al* (1993) Qa-2 molecules are peptide receptors of higher stringency than ordinary class I molecules. *Nature* **361** 642

Townsend A and Bodmer HC (1989) Antigen recognition by class I-restricted T lymphocytes. *Annual Reviews of Immunology* **7** 601–624

Travers P, Blundell TL, Sternberg MJE and Bodmer WF (1984) Structural and evolutionary analysis of HLA-D-region products. *Nature* **310** 235–238

Wu M, Van Kaer L, Itchara S and Tonegawa S (1991) Highly restricted expression of the thymus leukaemia antigens on intestinal epithelial cells. *Journal of Experimental Medicine* **174** 213–218

The author is responsible for the accuracy of the references.

# MHC Class I–Peptide Interactions and TCR Recognition

**AIDEEN C M YOUNG[1,2] • WEIGUO ZHANG[2]**
**JAMES C SACCHETTINI[1] • STANLEY G NATHENSON[2]**
*[1]Department of Biochemistry; [2]Department of Microbiology and Immunology and Department of Cell Biology, Albert Einstein College of Medicine, Bronx, New York 10461*



## INTRODUCTION

One of the most enduring mysteries of cellular immunity concerns the strategies used by major histocompatibility complex (MHC) class I molecules for the selection of peptides as part of the process of MHC restriction. In this process, peptide fragments of endogenously synthesized proteins associate with MHC class I molecules in the endoplasmic reticulum (Townsend *et al,* 1985). The complex that results is then transported to the cell surface for appraisal by the T cell receptors (TCR) of cytotoxic T lymphocytes (CTL) (Zinkernagel and Doherty, 1979; Townsend *et al,* 1985; Falk *et al,* 1990, 1991a; Van Bleek and Nathenson, 1990). If the peptide that is presented is recognized by the TCR as having been derived from a virus, tumour cell or other intracellular pathogen, processes leading to cell lysis are triggered (Zinkernagel and Doherty, 1979; Townsend *et al,* 1989). A given individual possesses three to six different MHC class I molecules, and it has been estimated that a single MHC class I molecule is capable of binding upwards of 1000 different peptides (Hunt *et al,* 1992). Nevertheless, the set of peptides bound by a class I molecule is allele specific. Unravelling the mysteries of cellular immunity lies in understanding the remarkable allele specificity of MHC class I molecules

*Cancer Surveys* Volume 22: *Molecular Mechanisms of the Immune Response*

and how high affinity binding can be accomplished with a large number and variety of peptides.

Class I molecules are encoded by a cluster of closely linked genes that are characterized by their extraordinary polymorphism (Trowsdale and Campbell, 1992). The protein encoded by the MHC is a glycoprotein consisting of a polymorphic heavy chain with a molecular mass of 45 kDa non-covalently associated with the invariant light chain, $\beta_2$ microglobulin (B2M) whose molecular mass is 11 kDa. The heavy chain consists of three distinct portions: cytoplasmic, transmembrane and extracellular, the latter being composed of the $\alpha$1, $\alpha$2 and $\alpha$3 regions (Nathenson *et al,* 1981). The polymorphic residues are not randomly distributed throughout the molecule but have been found to be located mainly in $\alpha$1 and $\alpha$2 (Steinmetz and Hood, 1983; Nathenson *et al,* 1986).

That peptides constitute the antigenic epitope associated with class I molecules was demonstrated by Townsend and co-workers (1986) when they showed that a major part of the anti-influenza viral CTL response was directed towards peptides derived from influenza nucleoprotein. Many subsequent experiments similarly succeeded in showing that a class I directed immune response could be mimicked in vitro by short synthetic peptides added exogenously (Townsend *et al,* 1986; Gotch *et al,* 1987; Townsend and Bodmer, 1989). Although these synthetic peptides are associated with the MHC class I molecules, they do not necessarily have to be representative of antigens (foreign or self) that are processed endogenously (Fox *et al,* 1988; Bodmer *et al,* 1989). Hence, Van Bleek and Nathenson (1990) developed a method to isolate naturally processed ligands directly from class I molecules in the cell. Using a model system, they identified the major peptide epitope associated with the murine class I molecule H-2K$^b$ in vesicular stomatitis virus (VSV) infected cells, as an eight residue peptide derived from influenza nucleoprotein. Similarly, a nine residue peptide from influenza nucleoprotein was found to be H-2K$^d$ restricted (Rötzschke *et al,* 1990; Falk *et al,* 1991b). Extensive data from pool sequencing has now been amassed specifying the sequences of large numbers of peptides eluted from various human and murine class I molecules (Rammensee *et al,* 1993).

## ALLELE SPECIFIC PEPTIDE BINDING

Characterization of the naturally occurring peptides eluted from MHC class I molecules reveals that they are typically composed of eight or nine aminoacid residues (Rammensee *et al,* 1993). Furthermore, those bound to a single MHC class I allele all possess chemically similar residues at the C-terminal position of the peptide (denoted PC) and at least one other position along its length (denoted by P and the peptide residue position), and the identity of these consensus residues is allele specific (Rammensee *et al,* 1993). The conservation of the consensus or anchor residues suggested that they must be involved in the binding of the peptide to the MHC. Indeed, peptide variant studies have revealed that the replacement of any of the anchor residues Tyr3, Tyr5 or Leu8 of the VSV peptide by Ala completely abrogated binding to H-2K$^b$ (Shibata *et al*, 1992).

In peptides bound to H-2K$^b$, an aromatic residue (generally Tyr) is found at P5 and a hydrophobic residue (generally Leu) at PC (Falk *et al*, 1991a; Rötzschke *et al*, 1991; Schumacher *et al*, 1991; Van Bleek and Nathenson, 1991; Shiel *et al*, 1992). Peptides eluted from H-2D$^b$ show a preference for Asn at P5 and Met at P9 (Townsend *et al*, 1986; Kast *et al*, 1989; Falk *et al*, 1991a; Rötzschke *et al*, 1991). H-2K$^b$ and H-2D$^b$ differ from most of the murine and human class I molecules for which peptide motifs are known in that in addition to the anchor residue at PC of their bound peptides, they also have an anchor in the middle of the peptide sequence, as opposed to other murine and human class I molecules for which P2 is the additional peptide anchor position. Therefore, in the murine class I molecule H-2K$^d$, Tyr is found at P2 and Leu or Ile at PC (Maryanski *et al*, 1989, 1990; Romero *et al*, 1991). H-2K$^k$ shows a preference for Glu at P2 and Ile at PC (Gould *et al*, 1991; Cossins *et al*, 1993). In peptides bound to H-2L$^d$, Pro occurs preferentially at P2 and Leu at PC (Corr *et al*, 1992). Although there do not seem to be any restrictions on the identity of the second peptide anchor residue among all of the class I molecules, PC in the vast majority of epitopes is either Ile, Leu, Arg, Lys, Val, Tyr or Phe. In peptides bound to all murine class I molecules, this anchor residue is invariably hydrophobic (Falk *et al*, 1991a; Corr *et al*, 1992). In the H-2$^b$ mouse, Met is found for H-2D$^b$ and Leu for H-2K$^b$. By contrast, certain of the human MHC class I molecules, namely HLA-B27 and HLA-Aw68, bind peptides whose C-terminal anchor residue is Arg or Lys (Hunt *et al*, 1992). Although the anchor residue requirement is stringently imposed by an MHC molecule on potential epitopes, enormous degeneracy can be observed at all other peptide positions with no detriment to peptide binding.

Clearly, an understanding of the cellular immune response requires definition at a structural level of the properties of MHC class I molecules that determine the binding motifs, length and chemical and physical properties of the particular peptides presented as immunodominant epitopes.

## THE STRUCTURE OF THE MHC CLASS I MOLECULE

A significant step towards attaining this goal was achieved with the first X ray crystal structure determination of an MHC class I molecule, carried out in 1987 by Bjorkman *et al* (1987a,b) on the human class I molecule HLA-A2. This structure revealed that α1 and α2 together form one structural domain (α1/α2) supported by α3 and B2M (Fig. 1). The α1/α2 domain consists of two nearly anti-parallel α helices above a floor of eight β strands as shown in Fig. 1. Between the α helices lies a deep groove of approximately 25 Å long, 10 Å wide and 11 Å deep. The groove is in the most membrane distal portion of the

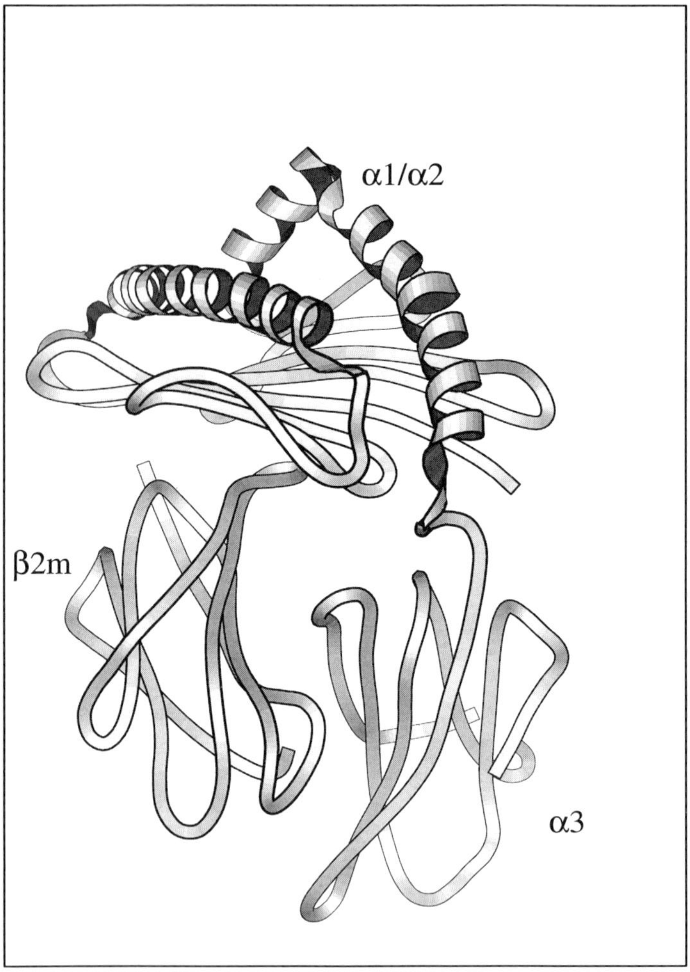


**Fig. 1.** Ribbon diagram of the backbone structure of the heavy chain and B2M of H-2D$^b$ (generated using MOLSCRIPT; Kraulis, 1991)

molecule and, were the complex cell bound, would be directed away from the cell surface in an ideal orientation for interaction with the TCR of a patrolling T cell. A large continuous region of electron density was located in this groove, and it was postulated that this density corresponded to the heterogeneous mixture of peptides that were present. These findings led to the hypothesis that the groove in the α1/α2 domain is the antigen binding site (Bjorkman *et al*, 1987a,b). Another intriguing feature revealed by analysis of the crystal structure was that the majority of the variable residues were located within the cleft. This strongly suggested that the particular combination and arrangement of variable residues serve to impart unique spatial and chemical characteristics to each cleft, which in turn dictate the properties of the peptides that bind.

Further gains in the study of MHC restriction would require the three dimensional structure determination of an MHC class I molecule with a homogeneous population of bound peptide. Only then, with the unambiguous assignment of the peptide residues, could it be definitively concluded that the antigen binding site is indeed located within the groove. Furthermore, examination of the precise interactions between single bound peptide and residues of the cleft would be necessary in order to elucidate the rules governing the selection of peptide epitopes.

## STRUCTURES OF MHC CLASS I MOLECULES WITH SINGLE ANTIGENIC PEPTIDES: STRATEGIES FOR PEPTIDE BINDING

The recent development of technology for the preparation and crystallization of MHC molecules containing single peptides has made possible the systematic examination of MHC complexes of different species (Fremont *et al,* 1992; Zhang *et al,* 1992; Young *et al,* 1994). The three dimensional structures of two murine class I molecules (H-2K$^b$ and H-2D$^b$) and a human (HLA-Aw68) MHC class I molecule containing single antigenic peptides have now been solved (Fremont *et al,* 1992; Silver *et al,* 1992; Zhang *et al,* 1992; Young *et al,* 1994). The crystal structure of recombinant, in vitro folded H-2D$^b$ containing a nine residue peptide from influenza nucleoprotein (Np366–374) (ASNENMETM) from influenza virus strain A/PR/8/34 has been solved and refined to 2.4 Å resolution (Fig. 2A). The structure of H-2K$^b$ has been solved containing both a single eight residue peptide (Fig. 2B) from VSV (RGYVYQGL) (Zhang *et al,* 1992) and a nine residue peptide (FAPGNYPAL), SEV-9, from Sendai virus nucleoprotein (Fremont *et al,* 1992). The crystal structure of the human class I molecule HLA-Aw68 has been solved with a nine residue peptide (KTGGPIYKR) from influenza virus nucleoprotein (Silver *et al,* 1992). The overall backbone structures of the recombinant H-2D$^b$, H-2K$^b$ and HLA complexes are very similar (Bjorkman *et al,* 1987a,b; Madden *et al,* 1992; Silver *et al,* 1992; Zhang *et al,* 1992; Young *et al,* 1994) as expected from their high sequence identity. The greatest difference between H-2D$^b$ and H-2K$^b$ lies in the relative orientation of their heavy chain and B2M domains (Young *et al,* 1994), a finding that we propose is due to differences in four variable residues on the $\alpha1/\alpha2$ domain that make contacts with B2M in both structures. This observation concerning the differing orientation of B2M may be related to several reports concerning quantitative differences in the association of B2M with H-2K$^b$ and H-2D$^b$ (Boyd *et al,* 1992; Otten *et al,* 1992).

Comparison of these structures has permitted the determination of the rules for peptide binding. Since the two structures of H-2K$^b$ both contain peptides that differ in length by one aminoacid, we have learned how a given class I molecule can efficiently bind peptides of different lengths. An additional important reason for performing these studies arises because H-2K$^b$ and H-2D$^b$ are the only two known MHC class I molecules in mice of the H-2$^b$ haplotype that present peptides to CD8 positive T cells. Analysis of their structures therefore provided the opportunity to understand the structural basis of antigen determinant selection in the cytotoxic T cell mediated immune response of this widely studied mouse.

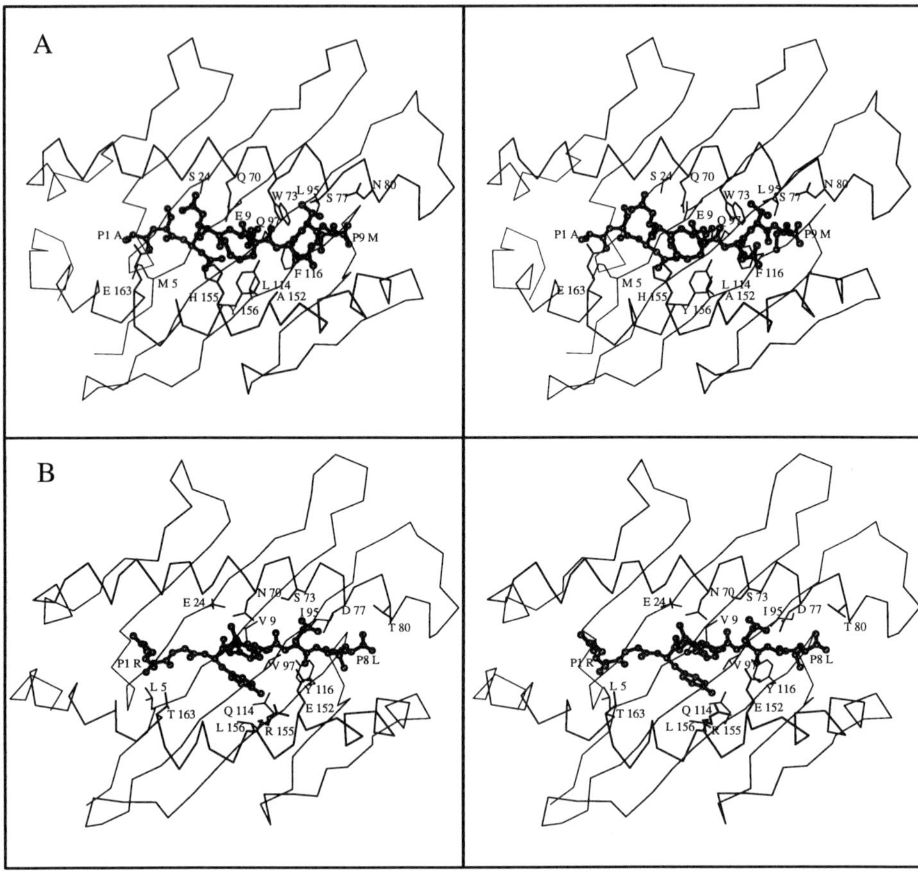


**Fig. 2.** Stereodiagram of the α-carbon trace of the antigen presenting domain of H-2D$^b$ (A) and of H-2K$^b$ (B). The side chains of those 15 cleft residues that differ between the two molecules are also shown. Of those 15 residues in H-2D$^b$, W73, L95, L114, F116, A152 and M5 are non-polar; S24, Q70, S77, Q97, N80 and Y156 are polar; and E9, H155 and E163 are ionizable. In H-2K$^b$ L5, V9, I95, V97 and L156 are non-polar; N70, S73, T80, Y116, Q114 and T163 are polar and E24, D77, E152 and R155 are ionizable. Both peptides are shown in ball and stick representations: the influenza peptide in (A) and the VSV peptide in (B). (Reproduced with the permission of *Cell Press* from Young *et al*, 1994)

## How is the Bound Peptide Held in the Groove?

The crystal structures of H-2D$^b$ with the nine residue influenza virus peptide (Young *et al*, 1994), H-2K$^b$ with both the eight residue VSV peptide (Zhang *et al*, 1992) and the nine residue SEV-9 peptide (Fremont *et al*, 1992) and HLA-Aw68 with the nine residue peptide Np91–99 (Silver *et al*, 1992) all show the peptide bound in a strikingly similar orientation. Superposition of the main chain atoms of the heavy chains of H-2K$^b$ and H-2D$^b$ shows that the VSV, SEV-9 and influenza peptides are highly superimposable, both for their main chain atoms and in the orientations of their side chains (Fig. 3). Each peptide is bound in a mostly extended conformation, maintained through a large number of hydrogen bonds between the peptide and residues of the cleft (Table 1).

A

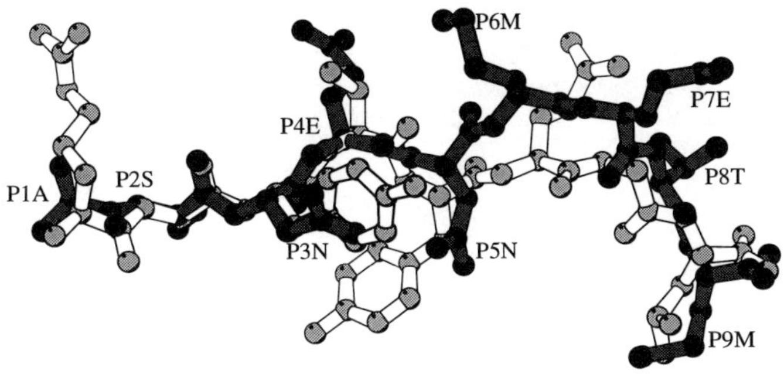


B

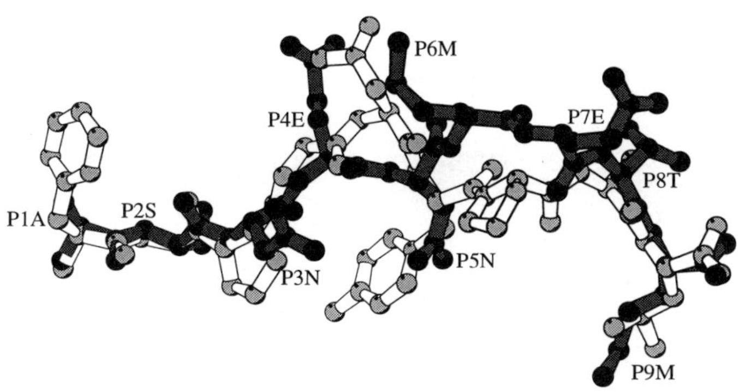


**Fig. 3.** (A) Sideview of the influenza peptide (filled circles, dark bonds) overlaid on the VSV peptide (shaded circles, white bonds), and (B), on the SEV-9 peptide (shaded circles, white bonds), obtained by superimposing the heavy chains of H-2D$^b$ and H-2K$^b$. Labelled residues are those of the influenza peptide. (Fig. 3A reproduced with the permission of *Cell Press* from Young *et al*, 1994)

Despite differences in the length and composition of the peptides, the distance between their termini as they lie in the cleft is approximately a constant (Fig. 3). This distance is 24.76 Å for the influenza derived peptide in H-2D$^b$, 24.96 Å for the eight-residue VSV peptide bound to H-2K$^b$ and 25.4 Å for the SEV-9 peptide bound to H-2K$^b$. The constancy of this distance is an important feature in MHC class I peptide binding and is a consequence of conserved hydrogen bonding networks between the peptide termini and residues of the cleft that act to tether the ends of the peptide, thereby placing it in the cleft in the proper orientation. The conserved length of the bound peptide is also a consequence of the bulky conserved residues of the class I MHC that serve to block off the end of the binding cleft (Fig. 4). This is in contrast to the MHC class II structure where no such bulky residues are found, causing the peptide binding groove to extend much further than its class I counterpart and giving

**TABLE 1. Hydrogen bonds between bound peptide and residues of the cleft in the H-2D$^b$ influenza peptide complex, the H-2K$^b$ VSV peptide complex and the H-2K$^b$ SEV-9 peptide complex**

| Influenza | H-2D$^b$ | VSV | H-2K$^b$ | SEV-9 | H-2K$^b$ |
|---|---|---|---|---|---|
| P1A N | OH-Y171 | P1R N | OH-Y171 | P1F N | OH-Y171,OH-Y7 |
| O | OH-Y159 | O | OH-Y159 | O | OH-Y159 |
| P2S N | OE2-E63 | P2G N | OE1,OE2-E63 | P2A N | OE1-E63 |
| O | NZ-K66 | O | NZ-K66 | O | NZ-K66 |
| OG | OE2-E63 | | | | |
| | OH-Y45[a] | | | | |
| | OH-Y22[a] | | | | |
| P3N N | OG-S99[a] | P3Y O | ND2-N70 | P3P N | |
| | | | | O | ND2-N70,OE2-E24[a] |
| OD1 | OE1-E9[a] | | | | |
| | NE2-Q70 | | | | |
| P4E O | NE2-H155 | | | | |
| P5N N | OE1-Q70 | P5Y N | OE1-N70 | P5N N | OD1-N70[a] |
| ND2 | OH-Y156 | | | | |
| OD1 | NE2-Q97 | | | | |
| | | | | P6Y N | OD1-N70[a] |
| P6M O | NE1-W73 | P6E O | NE1-W147 | O | OH-S73 |
| SD | ND1-H155 | | | OH | O-Y7[a],OE2-E24[a] |
| | | | | | OH-S99[a] |
| P7E O | NE1-W73 | P7G O | OE1,OE2-D77 | | |
| OE1 | OG-S150 | | | | |
| P8T O | NE1-W147 | P8L O | OH-Y84, | P8A O | NE1-W147 |
| | | | OD1-T143 | | |
| | | OT | OD1-T80 | | |
| | | | | P9L N | OD2-D77, |
| | | | | | OD1-T80[a] |
| P9M O | ND2-N80 | | | P9L O | OH-Y84,OD1-T143 |
| OT | OH-Y84 | | | P9L OT | NZ-K146, |
| | OG1-T143 | | | | OD1-T80[a], |
| | | | | | OD2-D77[a] |

[a]Hydrogen bonds mediated by a water molecule
P = position

rise to the binding of much longer peptides (Brown *et al*, 1993). It is significant that the majority of the variable residues that map into the antigen binding groove are located along its length, whereas those residues whose function is to block the ends of the groove and hydrogen bond to the peptide termini are highly conserved (Fig. 4).

The main chain N and O atoms of P1 of VSV, SEV-9, Np91–99 and the influenza derived peptide all form hydrogen bonds with the hydroxyl groups of Tyr159 and Tyr171 at the end of the groove (Table 1) (Fremont *et al*, 1992; Silver *et al*, 1992; Zhang *et al*, 1992; Young *et al*, 1994). In addition, the main chain N atoms of SEV-9 and Np91–99 hydrogen bond with Y7. These hydrogen bonds orient the peptide such that its terminal N atom points towards the floor of the cleft with the result that the side chain at position P1 of the peptide is directed out of the cleft (Fig. 3). Since the side chain of P1 points outwards, it may explain why a relatively high level of degeneracy is ob-

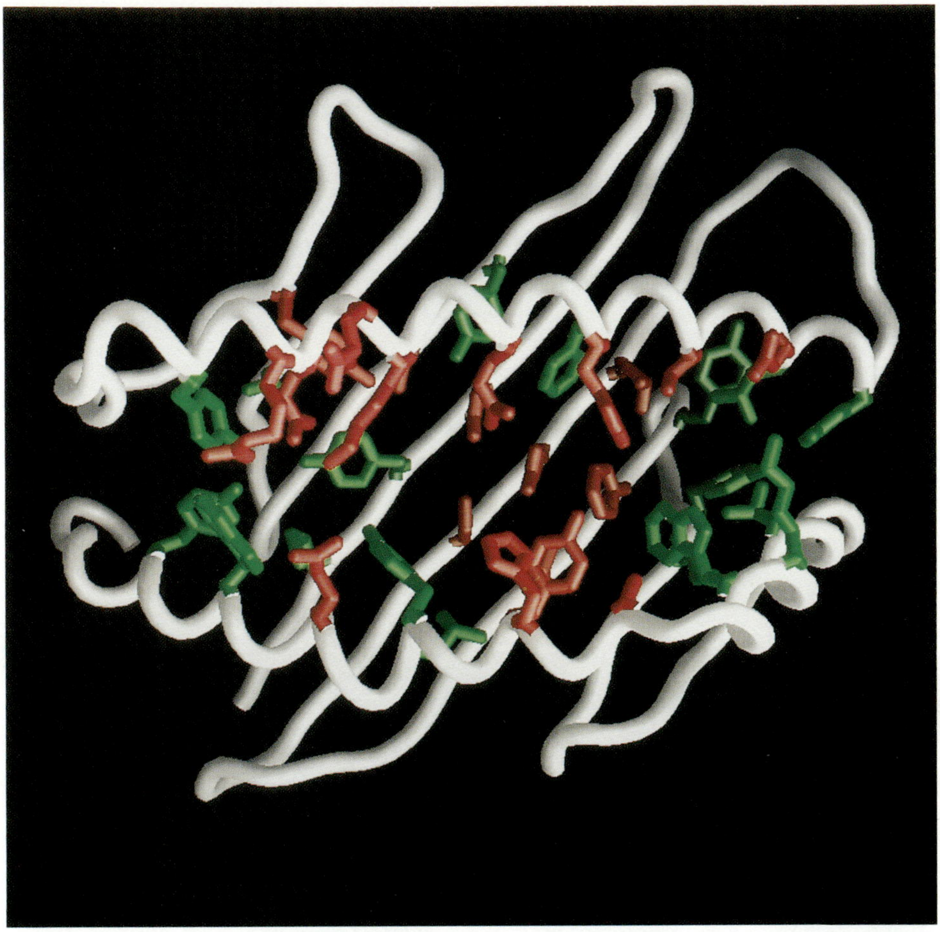

**Fig. 4.** Backbone trace of the antigen presenting domain of H-2D$^b$ with the side chains of cleft residues that are conserved and those that are variable among all murine class I molecules shown in green and red, respectively (generated with GRASP)

served at this position. At their C-termini, each peptide forms hydrogen bonding interactions with the conserved cleft residues Tyr84 and Thr143 and with residue 80 (Table 1). These residues are less buried than the cleft residues that are involved in hydrogen bonding the N-terminus. To maintain these hydrogen bonding interactions, the peptide must be oriented so that the side chain of its terminal aminoacid is buried and its carboxyl group is exposed on the surface of the cleft. These same hydrogen bonding interactions have been deduced for the structure of a complex of the human class I molecule HLA-B27 with a heterogeneous population of bound peptides (Madden *et al,* 1992). There is ample evidence then that the hydrogen bonding networks between the bound peptide and conserved residues at both ends of the cleft are themselves conserved. They tether the ends of the peptide in the cleft, fixing the positions of the peptide termini and restricting the lengths of peptides that will bind to the MHC.

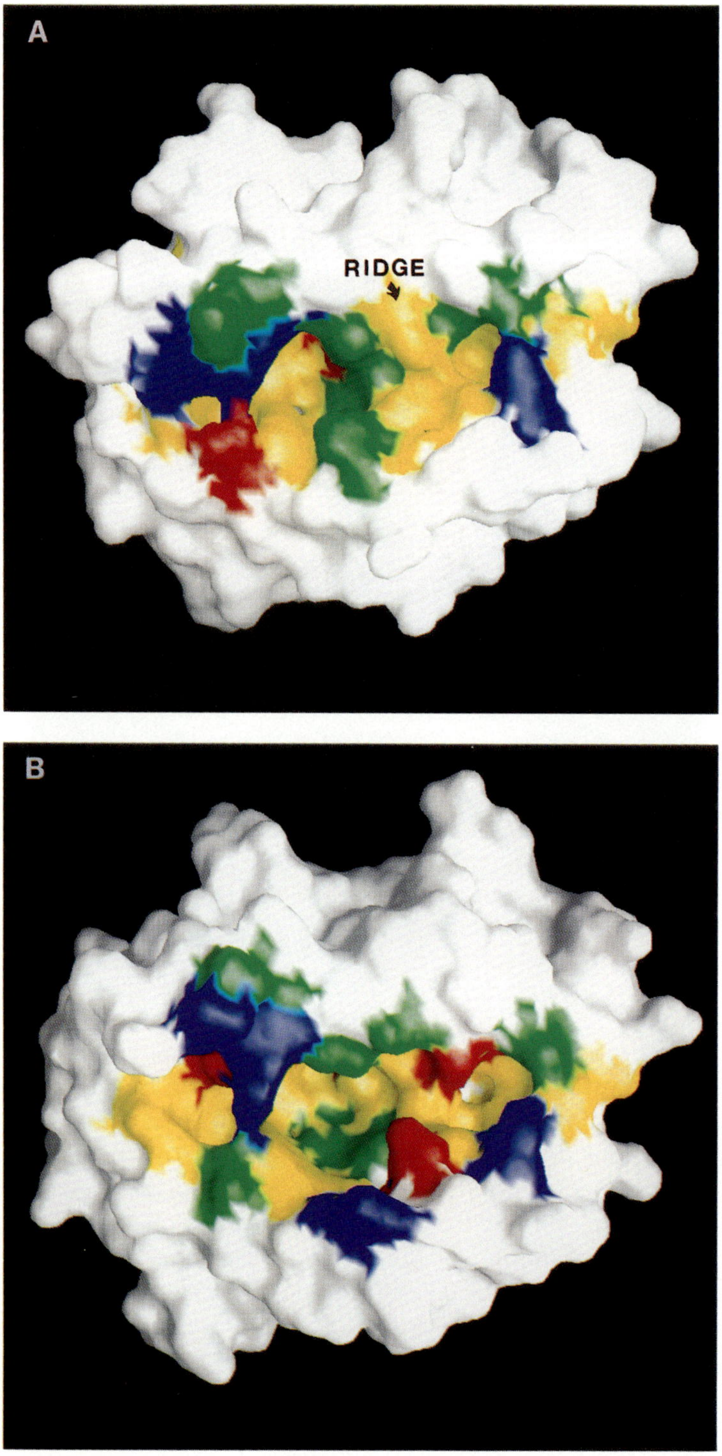


**Fig. 5.** *(See facing page for legend.)*

In addition to the hydrogen bonds involving the N- and C-termini of the peptide, other hydrogen bonds along the length of the bound peptide serve to hold it in the groove (Table 1). These hydrogen bonds are overwhelmingly between side chain atoms of residues lining the cleft and backbone atoms of the peptide. In the case of the VSV peptide bound in H-2K$^b$, all of its hydrogen bonding interactions involve its main chain atoms (Zhang *et al,* 1992); in the case of the SEV-9 peptide bound in H-2K$^b$ (Fremont *et al,* 1992), only P6Tyr makes side chain hydrogen bonds, although they are not direct, being mediated by an ordered solvent molecule. The influenza peptide bound to H-2D$^b$ (Young *et al,* 1994) makes a total of 22 hydrogen bonds with atoms of the cleft, and only the side chains of P2Ser and P5Asn make direct hydrogen bonds with cleft residues.

Among murine class I allelic products, all of the cleft residues that hydrogen bond to the bound peptide, with the exception of those that hydrogen bond to the peptide termini as well as Trp147, are variable (Young *et al,* 1994). Nevertheless, the side chains of the same ten cleft residues were used in hydrogen bonding to the peptide in both the H-2D$^b$- and the H-2K$^b$-VSV complexes, and nine of those cleft residues also hydrogen bond to the SEV-9 peptide when bound to H-2K$^b$ (Table 1). Hence, conserved hydrogen bonding networks exist to bind the peptide in the cleft, and these networks use not only the conserved residues at the ends of the cleft, but also certain variable residues positioned throughout it. As the majority of the hydrogen bonds between the bound peptide and residues of the cleft use the main chain atoms of the peptide, a very large number of peptides (of the appropriate length) can be accommodated in a given cleft. The hydrogen bonding schemes employed in the class I structures explain the enormous degeneracy observed in peptide binding.

## The Properties of the Antigen Binding Cleft Give Rise to an Allele Specific Motif

Of the 180 residues in the α1/α2 domain of the H-2D$^b$ and H-2K$^b$ molecules, 36 contribute atoms to the molecular surface of the peptide binding groove (Young *et al,* 1994). Of these residues, 21 are identical between D$^b$ and K$^b$ and are in very similar conformations in both structures. The composition of the 15 variable residues, which provide the diversity in the properties of the cleft, is very similar between the two molecules (Fig. 2). In H-2D$^b$, six of these 15 var-

**Fig. 5.** Surface representation (using GRASP) of the antigen presenting domains of H-2D$^b$ (A) and of H-2K$^b$ (B). The surface of hydrophobic residues (Gly, Ala, Val, Ile, Leu, Phe, Pro, Met, Trp, Tyr) is yellow; of polar residues (Cys, Ser, Thr, Asn, Gln, His) green; of positively charged residues (Lys and Arg) blue; and of negatively charged residues (Asp and Glu) red. The hydrophobic ridge of the H-2D$^b$ cleft is indicated. The orientation of the cleft is identical in both panels—a peptide would bind such that its N-terminus would be at the leftmost end and its C-terminus at the rightmost end of the cleft as shown

iable residues are non-polar, six are polar and three are ionizable, whereas in H-2K$^b$, five are non-polar, six are polar and four are ionizable. The 15 variable residues in the H-2K$^d$ cleft are made up of six non-polar, five polar and four charged residues. In H-2K$^k$, they are instead made up of three non-polar, six polar and six charged residues. Thus, the identity of the variable residues in an allele and their distribution within its cleft convey upon that cleft its own distinctive set of steric and chemical properties.

### *The Effects on Peptide Length*

Although the hydrogen bonding networks with conserved residues at both ends of the cleft control the approximate lengths of peptides that bind (eight or nine residue peptides), mid-cleft architecture is also a factor. The most distinctive feature in the H-2D$^b$ cleft is caused by Trp73 on the α1 helix and Tyr156 on the α2 helix (Ser73 and Leu156 in H-2K$^b$) (Young *et al,* 1994). The side chains of Trp73 and Tyr156 point towards one another across the groove, and along with the side chain of Trp147 on the α2 helix, which is conserved in all MHC class I molecules, form a hydrophobic ridge between the α1 and α2 helices that runs nearly perpendicular to the long axis of the cleft (Fig. 5). The H-2K$^d$ molecule also has Trp at position 73 and Tyr at 156, and modelling studies have confirmed the existence of a prominent hydrophobic ridge in this allele as well. The structure of H-2D$^b$ revealed that the bound peptide is forced to rise over the Trp73-Tyr156-Trp147 ridge in the floor of the cleft, causing a pronounced arch in the peptide backbone from P5 to P7 (Fig. 3). H-2D$^b$, H-2K$^d$ and other alleles that possess this structural feature would not be expected to be able to bind peptides that have fewer than nine residues. H-2K$^b$ accommodates the nine residue SEV-9 peptide by forming a kink in the peptide backbone at positions P4 and P5 (Fig. 3), with the result that the aminoacids at these positions make no contacts with residues of the cleft (Fremont *et al,* 1992). A similar situation was described for HLA-Aw68 with Np91–99 (Silver *et al,* 1992). It has also been reported that even longer peptides (10 and 11 residue peptides) can bind to HLA-Aw68 by bulging out of the groove and into solvent (Guo *et al,* 1992). Thus, although the nine residue peptide bound in H-2D$^b$ was shown to maintain extensive hydrogen bonding and van der Waals' interactions along its length, the binding of longer peptides that kink outwards, making no contacts with residues of the groove, can also be tolerated. One might surmise, however, that such a situation would lead to peptides with lower binding affinities.

### *The Identity of the Anchor Residues*

Analysis of the MHC class I structures has revealed the structural basis for the anchor residue requirement. The precise steric and chemical properties of the cleft (Fig. 5) give rise to a unique peptide anchor motif. These structures show that each cleft consists of a series of depressions or indentations that serve to accommodate two or three side chains of the bound peptide (Garrett *et al,* 1989; Madden *et al,* 1991, 1992; Saper *et al,* 1991; Fremont *et al,* 1992; Matsumura *et al,* 1992; Zhang *et al,* 1992; Young *et al,* 1994). The invariability of the peptide termini among different complexes means that the side chains of different bound peptides occupy almost identical positions. The clefts of these different class I molecules can therefore be regarded as a set of peptide side chain binding sites, each of which has distinct features due to the variability among the residues of each cleft.

Figure 5 shows that the greatest differences between the H-2D$^b$ and H-2K$^b$ clefts occur from their mid-cleft regions through the ends of the groove corresponding to the C-terminal end of the $\alpha 1$ helix. Residues 9, 97 and 99 appear to be the primary determinants of the nature of this mid-cleft region. On the floor of the central portion of the K$^b$ cleft, the side chains of residues Val9, Val97 and Ser99 form a deep, spacious and hydrophobic depression. The X ray crystal structures of H-2K$^b$ with the VSV peptide (Zhang *et al,* 1992) and the SEV-9 peptide (Fremont *et al,* 1992) show that the anchor residue Tyr at P5 of both peptides is located in this central depression where it forms van der Waals' interactions with residues of the cleft. The corresponding region of the cleft in H-2D$^b$ has Glu9 (coloured red in Fig. 5), Gln97 and Ser99 (coloured green in Fig. 5) with the result that this part of the cleft is more shallow and polar in H-2D$^b$ than in H-2K$^b$ (Young *et al,* 1994). Nevertheless, this region of the D$^b$ cleft can accommodate Asn as the anchor residue at P5 of the bound peptide. Furthermore, the occurrence of Gln at position 97 clearly allows for a polar peptide anchor residue, and the crystal structure revealed that the side chain of P5Asn is hydrogen bonding with three cleft residues including Gln97.

As already noted, H-2K$^b$ and H-2D$^b$ are unique among class I molecules because one of their anchor residues occurs in the middle of the peptide sequence rather than at P2, the most common anchor residue position. Computer modelling of the clefts of other alleles quickly explains this predilection. H-2K$^d$ has Arg at position 97 and Phe at position 99; H-2K$^k$ also has Arg at position 97 and Tyr at 99 and H-2L$^d$ has Trp at 97 and Tyr at 99 (Corr *et al,* 1992). Thus, as a result of the presence of these bulky residues, H-2K$^d$, H-2K$^k$ and H-2L$^d$ have no depression in the central portion of their clefts and therefore no binding site for a central anchor residue. Rather, H-2K$^d$, H-2K$^k$ and H-2L$^d$, like most other alleles for which binding motifs are known, use a second anchor at P2 of the peptide.

The crystal structures of H-2K$^b$ and H-2D$^b$ have exposed the nature of the P2 binding site. It takes the form of a cavity in the wall of the cleft, beneath the $\alpha 1$ helix. This depression (often referred to as pocket B; Matsumura *et al,* 1992) is defined by residues 9, 24, 45, 67 and 99, and the identity of these residues determines the usage of this site. H-2K$^b$ is the least spacious of the alleles in this region of the cleft due to the occurrence of Tyr at position 45 and of Glu at 24. This is consistent with the fact that the VSV and SEV-9 peptides have Gly and Ala at position 2, respectively. The replacement of Glu at P24 of H-2K$^b$ by Ser in H-2D$^b$ allows for greater capacity in this region of the cleft, and in the structure of H-2D$^b$, P2Ser is directed into this cavity (Young *et al,* 1994). There is also sufficient space for an ordered water molecule with which the side chain of P2Ser is hydrogen bonding. In H-2K$^k$, the peptide motif calls for Glu at position P2 (Gould *et al,* 1991). Computer modelling shows that the P2 binding site in the H-2K$^k$ cleft is approximately the same size as that in H-2D$^b$ due to the fact that the cleft residues that contribute to this depression are roughly the same in both molecules. Presumably then, this site can equally well accommodate the side chain of a Ser residue plus a hydrogen bonded ordered solvent molecule or the side chain of Glu. This suggests that Ser at P2 of peptides binding to H-2D$^b$ is not a stringent requirement and that peptides whose P2 residue bears a longer side chain could also bind. Indeed, the sequencing of peptides eluted from H-2D$^b$ has not identified a consensus motif for the P2 peptide position. The presence of water molecules within the binding cleft is likely to be an important component of peptide binding schemes, allowing for greater variability in the choice of residues that can bind in a given site, and hence contributing to the enormous degeneracy observed. The presence of Ala at positions 24 and 67 of the H-2K$^d$ allele gives this molecule the largest P2 binding site, and computer modelling has confirmed that it is sufficiently large to accommodate Tyr as its preferred peptide anchor residue.

The side chain of the PC anchor residue in MHC class I molecules is located in a pocket where the cleft residues 74 and 116 are located. The chemical nature of these two residues appears to be critical in determining the identity of the C-terminal residue of the bound peptide. HLA-Aw68 binds peptides with Arg at PC forming a salt bridge with residues Asp74 and Asp116 (Silver *et al,* 1992). On the other hand, all the murine class I molecules bind peptides whose PC anchor residue is hydrophobic, generally Leu or Ile (Falk *et al,* 1991a; Corr *et al,* 1992). This is consistent with the finding that almost all of these molecules have Phe at position 74 and Tyr or Phe at position 116. Peptide binding in the MHC groove is therefore dependent on the existence of two principal peptide anchor residues whose position along the length of the peptide coincides with complimentary depressions in the cleft and whose physical and chemical properties must be compatible with those of the cleft.

## TCR RECOGNITION OF THE MHC-PEPTIDE COMPLEX

Analysis of the bound peptides in each of the crystal structures that has been discussed has identified those residues with high solvent accessibility. As these residues are directed out of the binding cleft, they are assumed to be available for contact by the TCR. In the case of the influenza peptide bound to H-2D$^b$, the side chains of residues P4Glu, P6Met and P7Glu all show high solvent accessibility (Fig. 3) (Young *et al,* 1994). That the side chains of these peptide residues are indeed involved in TCR interaction has been strongly suggested by earlier biological studies involving another naturally occurring antigenic peptide (ASNENMDAM) from the nucleoprotein of influenza isolate

A/NT/60/68, which differs from the Np366–374 peptide at positions P7 (E to D) and at P8 (T to A) (Bastin *et al,* 1987). It was found that this peptide and ASNENMETM are recognized in the context of H-2D$^b$ by one CTL clone, whereas recognition by a second CTL clone is completely abrogated by the single change from Asp to Glu at P7. These results suggested that the two peptides bind to H-2D$^b$ with similar conformations, not influenced by the identity of the residues at P7 or P8, and that these residues are instead interacting with the TCR. Similarly, amino acid substitution studies on another peptide presented by H-2D$^b$, the SV40 T antigen peptide (epitope I), implicate residues P6 to P8 as TCR contact residues (Deckhut and Tevethia, 1992). For peptides bound to H-2D$^b$, the side chains of P6 and P7 are solvent exposed because of the Trp73-Tyr156-Trp147 ridge that excludes their side chains from the interior of the cleft. Therefore, when peptides bind to MHC class I molecules that have Trp at position 73 and Tyr at position 156, we might therefore expect the peptide residues at P6 and P7 to be TCR contact residues.

In the case of the VSV peptide bound to H-2K$^b$, aminoacid substitution studies suggest that P1Arg, P4Val and P6Gln are the TCR contact residues (Shibata *et al,* 1992). The crystal structure has confirmed that the side chains of these residues are indeed the most solvent exposed (Zhang *et al,* 1992). By

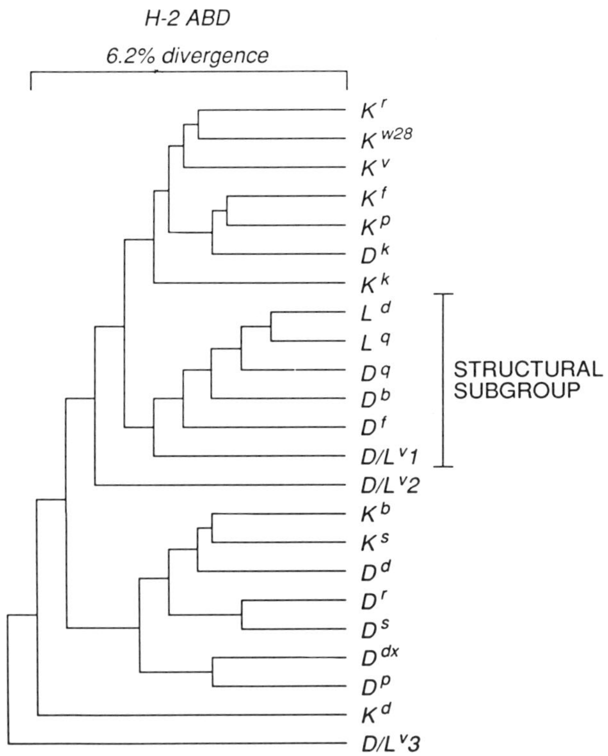


**Fig. 6.** Average distance tree of K, D and L sequences (reproduced with permission from Pullen *et al,* 1992, Copyright 1992, *The Journal of Immunology*). The structural subgroup is indicated

the same premise, the postulated TCR contact residues of the SEV-9 peptide bound in H-2K$^b$ are P1Arg, P4Gly, P5Tyr and P7Gln (Fig. 3) (Fremont *et al*, 1992). The extra contact residue in this peptide arises because the additional aminoacid causes a backbone kink at P4 and P5. The crystal structure of HLA-Aw68 with the Np91–99 peptide led to the conclusion that the peptide residues P1Lys, P4Gly, P5Pro, P6Ile, P7Tyr and P8Lys may all be available for TCR contact (Silver *et al*, 1992).

The TCR therefore contacts a composite structure comprising several exposed side chains of the bound peptide and residues on the MHC class I molecule itself. Fremont *et al* (1992) found small conformational differences in the structure of H-2K$^b$ as a result of binding two different peptides and suggested that these subtle synergistic movements by the protein molecule on peptide binding may be an intrinsic aspect of the recognition process.

## A SUBCLASS OF MHC CLASS I ALLELES HAS A CONSERVED STRUCTURAL FEATURE

The occurrence of Trp at position 73 in molecules of the D series is always accompanied by Tyr at position 156. This is observed to be the case for D$^b$, D$^f$, D$^q$, D$^{lvl}$ as well as for L$^d$ and L$^q$, which are thought to be closely related to the D series, and for a single allele of the K series, K$^d$. These seven molecules therefore all possess the hydrophobic ridge that has been discussed. It is of interest in this regard that both H-2K$^d$ (Falk *et al*, 1991a,b) and L$^d$ (Corr *et al*, 1992) have been shown to bind nine residue peptides, which is the minimal length peptide expected to bind to H-2D$^b$ as a result of the ridge (Young *et al*, 1994). As the ridge containing molecules represent approximately 25% of the murine class I molecules whose sequences have been reported (Pullen *et al*, 1992), these molecules were classified as a structural subclass (Young *et al*, 1994). The Trp73-Tyr156-Trp147 ridge is peculiar to the mouse and is not found in any of the human class I alleles. This subdivison based on a distinctive structural feature correlates well with evolutionary studies on murine class I molecules, as shown in Fig. 6. This average distance tree, calculated for the antigen presenting domain of K and D/L sequences (reproduced with permission from Pullen *et al*, 1992), shows the evolutionary relationship of these alleles. The six D/L alleles that possess the Trp73-Tyr156-Trp147 ridge appear from this analysis to have evolved from a common progenitor and are more similar than any other group of mouse alleles. It appears, then, that the six D/L proteins are related to one another by random locus specific mutations, indicating an evolutionary pressure to conserve the ridge within this group or subclass of MHCs. The members of this subclass have therefore evolved in a classical fashion, in a manner similar to that of alleles of the HLA system, in contrast to the antigen presenting domains of the remaining K and D/L alleles, which do not show significant clustering. It is intriguing to speculate whether further MHC class I peptide structures might reveal structural features specific to a particular species. Such a finding would indicate that certain structural features at the protein level control the natural selection of genes diversified by point mutations and by recombinant mechanisms such as microgene conversion.

## SUMMARY

The recent crystal structure determinations of MHC class I molecules with single bound peptides have allowed us to understand the guidelines that govern peptide binding in a given MHC allele. Evolution has provided for MHC class I molecules whose antigen binding clefts possess distinct physical and chemical properties as a result of the particular arrangement of variable residues lining the binding cleft. As a result, a given molecule binds a unique set of peptides, the position and identity of whose anchor residues are dictated by the features of the cleft. In addition to the interactions between the anchor residues and the cleft, the peptide is held in the groove by a highly conserved array of hydrogen bonds. A tantalizing application of our newfound understanding of peptide binding will be in the design of model peptides that either block or enhance immune response, in order to achieve effective treatments for a variety of disorders of the immune system.

## Acknowledgements

We thank A Nicholls and B Honig for the use of their programme GRASP. Many thanks also to Cole Thomson for help with the modelling. This work was supported by National Institutes of Health grants 5 R37 AI-07289, 1RO1 GM-45859, 2PO1 AI-10792, 2 P30 CA-13330 and 1 RO1 AI-27199. ACMY is supported by a postdoctoral fellowship from the Irvington Institute for Medical Research.

## References

Bastin J, Rothbard J, Davey J, Jones I and Townsend A (1987) Use of synthetic peptides of influenza nucleoprotein to define epitopes recognized by class I-restricted cytotoxic T lymphocytes. *Journal of Experimental Medicine* **165** 1508–1523

Bjorkman PJ, Saper MA, Samraoui B, Bennett WS, Strominger JL and Wiley DC (1987a) Structure of the human class I histocompatibility antigen HLA-A2. *Nature* **329** 506–512

Bjorkman PJ, Saper MA, Samraoui B, Bennett WS, Strominger JL and Wiley DC (1987b) The foreign antigen binding site and T cell recognition regions of class I histocompatibility antigens. *Nature* **329** 512–518

Bodmer HC, Gotch FM and McMichael AJ (1989) Class I cross-restricted T cells reveal low responder allele due to processing of viral antigen. *Nature* **337** 653–655

Boyd LF, Kozlowski S and Margulies DH (1992) Solution binding of an antigenic peptide to a major histocompatibility complex class I molecule and the role of $\beta_2$-microglobulin. *Im-*

*munology* **89** 2242–2246

Brown JH, Jardetzky TS, Gorga JC *et al* (1993) Three-dimensional structure of the human class II histocompatibility antigen HLA-DR1. *Nature* **364** 33–39

Corr M, Boyd LF, Frankel SR, Kozlowski S, Padlan EA and Margulies DH (1992) Endogenous peptides of a soluble major histocompatibility complex class I molecule, H-2$L^d_s$: sequence motif, quantitative binding, and molecular modeling of the complex. *Journal of Experimental Medicine* **176** 1681–1692

Cossins J, Gould KG, Smith M, Driscoll P and Brownlee GG (1993) Precise prediction of a $K^k$-restricted cytotoxic T cell epitope in the NS1 protein of influenza virus using an MHC allele-specific motif. *Virology* **193** 289–295

Deckhut AM and Tevethia SS (1992) Effect of point mutations in the native simian virus-40 tumor antigen, and in the synthetic peptides corresponding to the H-2D(b)-restricted epitopes, on antigen presentation and recognition by cytotoxic lymphocyte-T clones. *Journal of Immunology* **148** 3012–3020

Falk K, Rötzschke O and Rammensee H-G (1990) Cellular peptide composition governed by major histocompatibility complex class I molecules. *Nature* **348** 248–250

Falk K, Rötzschke O, Stevanovic S, Jung G and Rammensee H-G (1991a) Allele-specific motifs revealed by sequencing of self-peptides eluted from MHC molecules. *Nature* **351** 290–296

Falk K, Rötzschke O, Deres K, Metzger J, Jung G and Rammensee H-G (1991b) Identification of naturally processed viral nonapeptides allows their quantification in infected cells and suggests an allele-specific T cell epitope forecast. *Journal of Experimental Medicine* **174** 425–434

Fox BS, Carbone FR, Germain RN, Paterson Y and Schwartz RH (1988) Processing of a minimal antigenic peptide alters its interaction with MHC molecules. *Nature* **331** 538–540

Fremont DH, Matsumura M, Stura EA, Peterson PA and Wilson IA (1992) Crystal structures of two viral peptides in complex with murine MHC class I H-2$K^b$. *Science* **257** 919–927

Garrett TPJ, Saper MA, Bjorkman PJ, Strominger JL and Wiley DC (1989) Specificity pockets for the side chains of peptide antigens in HLA-Aw68. *Nature* **342** 692–696

Gotch FM, Rothbard J, Howland K, Townsend ARM and McMichael A (1987) Cytotoxic T lymphocytes recognize a fragment of influenza virus matrix protein in association with HLA-A2. *Nature* **326** 881–882

Gould KG, Scotney H and Brownlee GG (1991) Characterization of two distinct major histocompatibility complex class I $K^k$-restricted T-cell epitopes within the influenza A/PR/8/34 virus hemagglutinin. *Journal of Virology* **65** 5401–5409

Guo H-C, Jardetzky TS, Garrett TPJ, Lane WS, Strominger JL and Wiley DC (1992) Different length polypeptides bind to HLA-Aw68 similarly at their ends but bulge out in the middle. *Nature* **360** 364–366

Hunt DF, Henderson RA, Shabanowitz J *et al* (1992) Characterization of peptides bound to the class I MHC molecule HLA-A2.1 by mass spectrometry. *Science* **255** 1261–1263

Kast WM, Offringa R, Peters PJ *et al* (1989) Eradication of adenovirus E1-induced tumors by E1A-specific cytotoxic T lymphocytes. *Cell* **59** 603–614

Kraulis PJ (1991) MOLSCRIPT: a program to produce both detailed and schematic plots of protein structures. *Journal of Applied Crystallography* **24** 946–950

Madden DR, Gorga J, Strominger JL and Wiley DC (1991) The structure of HLA-B27 reveals nonamer self peptides bound in an extended conformation. *Nature* **353** 321–325

Madden DR, Gorga JC, Strominger JL and Wiley DC (1992) The three-dimensional structure of HLA-B27 at 2.1 Å resolution suggests a general mechanism for tight peptide binding to MHC. *Cell* **70** 1035–1048

Maryanski JL, Abastado J-P, Corradin G and Cerottini J-C (1989) Structural features of peptides recognized by H-2$K^d$-restricted T cells. *Cold Spring Harbor Symposia in Quantitative Biology* **54** 545–550

Maryanski JL, Verdini AS, Weber PC, Salemme FR and Corradin G (1990) Competitor analogs for defined T cell antigens: peptides incorporating a putative binding motif and polyproline or polyglycine spacers. *Cell* **60** 63–72

Matsumura M, Fremont DH, Peterson PA and Wilson IA (1992) Emerging principles for the recognition of peptide antigens by MHC class I molecules. *Science* **257** 927–934

Nathenson SG, Uehara H, Ewenstein BM, Kindt TJ and Coligan JE (1981) Primary structural analysis of transplantation antigens of the murine H-2 major histocompatibility complex. *Annual Review of Biochemistry* **50** 1025–1052

Nathenson SG, Geliebter J, Pfaffenbach GM and Zeff RA (1986) Murine major histocompatibility complex class I mutants: molecular analysis and structure-function implications. *Annual Review of Immunology* **4** 471–502

Otten GR, Bikoff E, Ribaudo RK, Kozlowski S, Margulies DH and Germain RN (1992) Peptide and $\beta_2$-microglobulin regulation of cell surface MHC class I conformation and expression. *Journal of Immunology* **148** 3723–3732

Pullen JK, Horton RM, Cai Z and Pease LR (1992) Structural diversity of the classical H-2 genes: K, D, and L. *Journal of Immunology* **148** 953–967

Rammensee H-G, Falk K and Rötzschke O (1993) MHC molecules as peptide receptors. *Current Opinion in Immunology* **5** 35–44

Rötzschke O, Falk K, Deres K *et al* (1990) Isolation and analysis of naturally processed viral peptides as recognized by cytotoxic T cells. *Nature* **348** 252–254

Rötzschke O, Falk K, Stevanovic S, Jung G, Walden P and Rammensee H-G (1991) Exact prediction of a natural T cell epitope. *European Journal of Immunology* **21** 2891–2894

Romero P, Corradin G, Luescher IF and Maryanski JL (1991) H-2K$^d$ restricted antigenic epitopes share a simple binding motif. *Journal of Experimental Medicine* **174** 603–612

Saper MA, Bjorkman PJ and Wiley DC (1991) Refined structure of the human histocompatibility antigen HLA-A2 at 2.6 Å resolution. *Journal of Molecular Biology* **219** 277–319

Schumacher TNM, De Bruijn MLH, Vernie LN *et al* (1991) Peptide selection by MHC class I molecules. *Nature* **350** 703–706

Shibata K-I, Imarai M, Van Bleek GM, Joyce S and Nathenson SG (1992) Vesicular stomatitis virus antigenic octapeptide N52-59 is anchored into the groove of the H-2K$^b$ molecule by the side chains of three amino acids and the main chain atoms of the amino terminus. *Proceedings of the National Academy of Sciences of the USA* **89** 3135–3139

Shiel JM, Shepherd SE, Klimo GF and Paterson Y (1992) Identification of an autologous insulin B chain peptide as a target for H-2K$^b$-restricted cytotoxic T lymphocytes. *Journal of Experimental Medicine* **175** 545–552

Silver ML, Guo H, Strominger JL and Wiley DC (1992) Atomic structure of a human MHC molecule presenting an influenza virus peptide. *Nature* **360** 367–369

Steinmetz M and Hood L (1983) Genes of the major histocompatibility complex in mouse and man. *Science* **222** 727–733

Townsend ARM and Bodmer H (1989) Antigen recognition by class I restricted T lymphocytes. *Annual Review of Immunology* **7** 601–624

Townsend ARM, Gotch FM and Davey J (1985) Cytotoxic T cells recognize fragments of the influenza nucleoprotein. *Cell* **42** 457–467

Townsend ARM, Rothbard J, Gotch FM, Bahadur G, Wraith D and McMichael AJ (1986) The epitopes of influenza nucleoprotein recognized by cytotoxic T lymphocytes can be defined with short synthetic peptides. *Cell* **44** 959–968

Townsend ARM, Ölén C, Bastin J, Ljunggren HG, Foster I and Kärre K (1989) Association of class I major histocompatibility heavy and light chains induced by viral peptides. *Nature* **340** 443–448

Trowsdale J and Campbell RD (1992) Complexity in the major histocompatibility complex. *European Journal of Immunogenetics* **19** 45–55

Van Bleek GM and Nathenson SG (1990) Isolation of an immunodominant viral peptide from the class I H-2K$^b$ molecule. *Nature* **348** 213–216

Van Bleek GM and Nathenson SG (1991) The structure of the antigen-binding groove of major histocompatibility complex class I molecules determines specific selection of self- peptides.

*Proceedings of the National Academy of Sciences of the USA* **88** 11032–11036

Young ACM, Zhang W, Sacchettini JC and Nathenson SG (1994) The three dimensional structure of H-2D$^b$ at 2.4 Å resolution: implications for antigen determinant selection. *Cell* **76** 39–50

Zhang W, Young ACM, Imarai M, Nathenson SG and Sacchettini JC (1992) Crystal structure of the major histocompatibility class I H-2K$^b$ molecule containing a single viral peptide: implications for peptide binding and T-cell receptor recognition. *Proceedings of the National Academy of Sciences of the USA* **89** 8403–8407

Zinkernagel RM and Doherty PC (1979) MHC-restricted cytotoxic T cells: studies on the biological role of polymorphic major transplantation antigens determining T cell restriction specificity, function and responsiveness. *Advances in Immunology* **27** 51–77

The authors are responsible for the accuracy of the references.

# Class I MHC–Peptide Interactions: Structural Requirements and Functional Implications

**HOWARD M GREY[1] • JÖRG RUPPERT[1] • ANTONELLA VITIELLO[1] JOHN SIDNEY[1] • W MARTIN KAST[2] • RALPH T KUBO ALESSANDRO SETTE**

[1]*Cytel, 3525 John Hopkins Court, San Diego, California 92121;* [2]*Department of Immunohematology and Bloodbank, University Hospital Leiden, 2300 RC Leiden, The Netherlands*



## INTRODUCTION

Presentation of endogenous antigenic peptides bound to major histocompatibility complex (MHC) molecules is a prerequisite for stimulation of a cytotoxic T cell response, thus representing a crucial defence mechanism against viral infections and certain tumours. A considerable amount of information on the details of this interaction has been provided by a series of structural studies, most importantly the solution of the three dimensional structure of the MHC class I molecules themselves (Bjorkman *et al,* 1987; Saper *et al,* 1991) and later the structure of class I–peptide complexes (Fremont *et al,* 1992). A series of studies led to the definition of a stringent size requirement for peptide binding to class I molecules (Rötzschke *et al,* 1990; Van Bleek and Nathenson, 1990; Cerundolo *et al,* 1991). Because of the homogeneity of size, it has been possible to identify class I allele specific motifs through the aminoacid sequence analysis of complex mixtures of naturally processed peptides eluted from class I molecules (Falk *et al,* 1991). According to these studies, peptides bound to class I molecules exhibit a typical length of 9±1 aminoacids and carry "anchor" residues crucial for binding, typically in position 2 and the C-terminal position.

*Cancer Surveys* Volume 22: *Molecular Mechanisms of the Immune Response*

The ability to identify the peptides that are capable of binding with high affinity to MHC molecules is of potential practical importance for the design of peptide based vaccines capable of generating cytotoxic T lymphocyte activity. To facilitate the identification of relevant peptides, in this chapter we describe (a) the peptide binding motifs for some of the most common human histocompatibility leucocyte antigen (HLA) alleles found in different ethnic human populations; (b) experiments to indicate that motifs define the great majority of peptides that, in fact, are capable of binding to the relevant MHC; (c) the role of secondary anchor residues in determining the MHC binding capacity of peptides; and (d) the correlation of binding affinity to MHC with immunogenicity of peptides.

## DEFINITION OF HLA-A ALLELE SPECIFIC MOTIFS FOR HLA-A*0101, A*0301, A*1101 AND A*2401

The studies of Rammensee and colleagues have shown that allele specific motifs for both murine and human class I MHC can be identified through the sequencing of peptide mixtures eluted from affinity purified class I molecules (Falk *et al,* 1991). These motifs are characterized in terms of peptide length (generally 9±1 aminoacid residues) and dominant aminoacids that occupy crucial positions in the peptide—that is, anchor residues.

In humans, HLA-A*0201 is expressed by a large proportion of individuals of various ethnic backgrounds (ranging from 25% in blacks to 54% among Chinese) (The Central Data Analysis Committee, 1991). However, since a significant fraction of the population does not express HLA-A*0201, the inclusion of four additional HLA alleles (HLA-A*0101, A*0301, A*1101 and A*2401) is required to cover a major proportion of many ethnic populations (The Central Data Analysis Committee, 1991). We initially sought to determine putative peptide motifs for these alleles using the approach described by Falk *et al* (1991). A summary of the motifs identified is presented in Table 1. Using this same approach in control experiments, we have also confirmed an HLA-A*0201 motif which is identical to that previously identified by Falk *et al* (1991); that is, anchor residues leucine (L) or methionine (M) were found at position 2, and valine (V) at the C-terminus, respectively, for peptides of nine or ten residues in length. For all the different alleles, although strong and weak residues as originally described by Falk *et al* (1991) could be identified at several other positions, since the differences were more modest and variable, these have been omitted from Table 1. In the case of HLA-A*0101, however, it appeared that a third anchor residue might be present at position 3. Thus, for this allele, two motifs were proposed: one with anchor residues at position 2 (threonine [T] or serine [S]) and at the C-terminus (tyrosine [Y]) for peptides of 9–10 residues, and the second motif with an anchor at position 3 (aspartic acid [D] or glutamic acid [E]), and at the C-terminus (Y). Alternatively, a motif with anchor positions at 2, 3 and the C-terminus was also considered possible.

**TABLE 1. Summary of HLA-A allele specific motifs**

| | Position | | | | | | | | |
|---|---|---|---|---|---|---|---|---|---|
| **Allele** | **1** | **2** | **3** | **4** | **5** | **6** | **7** | **8** | **9/10** |
| A*0101 | • | T,S | • | • | • | • | • | • | Y |
| A*0101 | • | • | D,E | • | • | • | • | • | Y |
| A*0201 | • | L,M | • | • | • | • | • | • | V |
| A*0301 | • | V,L,M | • | • | • | • | • | • | K |
| A*1101 | • | T,V | • | • | • | • | • | • | K |
| A*2401 | • | Y | • | • | • | • | • | • | F,L |

**TABLE 2. HLA-A motif anchor residues in polyalanine nonamers and decamers**

| | | Binding capacity (IC50 nM) | | | | |
|---|---|---|---|---|---|---|
| **Sequence** | **Motif** | **A*0101** | **A*0201** | **A*0301** | **A*1101** | **A*2401** |
| ATAKAAAAY | A1 | 15 | – | 329 | 77 | – |
| AADKAAAAY | A1 | 50 | – | – | – | – |
| ATDKAAAAY | A1 | 3 | – | 9250 | 840 | – |
| ALAKAAAAV | A2.1 | – | 125 | – | – | – |
| ALAAAAAAK | A3 | – | – | 85 | 33 | – |
| ATAAAAAAK | A11 | – | – | 59 | 40 | – |
| AYAKAAAAF | A24 | – | – | – | – | 115 |

A dash indicates an IC50% (50% inhibitory concentration) greater than 10 000 nM

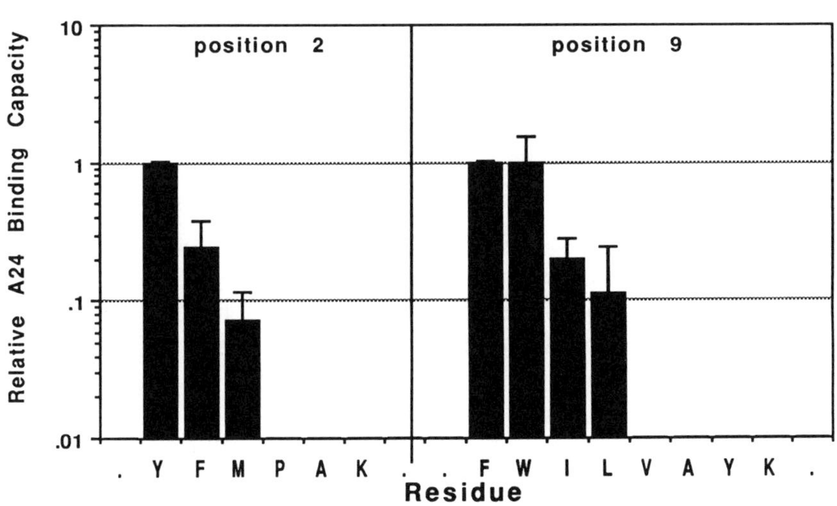


**Fig. 1.** HLA-A*2401 binding of polyalanine analogues. Single aminoacid substitutions of the parental polyalanine nonamer peptide, AYAKAAAAF, were tested for binding to purified HLA-A*2401 molecules. The indicated residues were introduced at anchor positions 2 and 9. Binding is expressed relative to the parental unsubstituted peptide

Interestingly, the HLA-A*1101 motif was very similar to the one obtained for HLA-A*0301. More specifically, the putative motif was defined by the presence of T or V anchor residues at position 2 for HLA-A*1101 and by V, L or M for HLA-A*0301. At the C-terminus, K defined the second anchor residue for both HLA-A*0301 and HLA-A*1101. Finally, for HLA-A*2401, the motif was characterized for peptides of 9–10 residues as having a Y as the anchor residue in position 2 and a phenylalanine (F) or L residue at the C-terminal positions.

## VALIDATION OF HLA-A ALLELE SPECIFIC PEPTIDE MOTIFS

We have recently established class I–peptide binding assays in solution based on the technology developed to analyse class II–peptide interactions and on the knowledge derived from the definition of the class I allele specific peptide motifs (Falk *et al,* 1991; Sette *et al,* 1991). We have used these quantitative peptide binding assays to verify the correctness of the motifs derived from the aminoacid sequence data from the peptide pools and to determine whether other residues that were not identified from the pooled peptide sequencing analysis could also serve as anchors. For this approach, peptides were synthesized with specific HLA-A motifs—that is, anchor residues embedded in a neutral backbone composed of alanine residues. The use of such "neutral" polyalanine (poly[A]) backbones as applied to the case of class II molecules has been described in detail (Jardetzky *et al,* 1990; Sette *et al,* 1992). In some of the peptides, a lysine residue was introduced within the sequence for the purpose of increasing peptide solubility. The results of the binding analysis of these poly(A) peptides are shown in Table 2. In all cases, the presence of the specific HLA-A motif anchor residues was sufficient to permit binding of the peptide to the relevant HLA-A allele product. Estimated $k_D$ values ranged from 3 to 125 nmol.

To address the issue of whether other chemically related aminoacids might also be tolerated in the crucial anchor positions, additional polyalanine analogues were synthesized by varying the residues present in position 2, 3 or 9. The peptides were then evaluated for binding to the appropriate HLA-A alleles. An example of this analysis for HLA-A*2401 is shown in Fig. 1. In this case, only a phenylalanine residue could serve as an alternative for tyrosine at position 2, with M yielding a weaker binding peptide. At the C-terminal position, tryptophan was equivalent to F as an anchor, and both leucine and isoleucine were found to be acceptable anchor residues. Indeed, the presence of a leucine at the C-terminal position was also deduced from the analysis of the pooled peptide sequencing data.

Similar studies were performed with HLA-A*0101, A*0201, A*0301 and A*1101. On the basis of these and other results (Kast *et al,* 1994; Kubo *et al,* 1994), we propose a refinement of the motifs for the different HLA-A alleles to include alternative anchor residues that were not predicted from the pooled sequencing data. These expanded HLA-A motifs are given in Table 3.

**TABLE 3. Expanded HLA-A allele specific motifs**

| Allele | Position 2 | Position 9 or 10 |
|---|---|---|
| A*0101 | T, S, M[a] | Y |
| A*0201 | L, M, (I, V, A, T)[b] | L, V, I, (A, M)T[c] |
| A*0301 | L, M, I, V, S, A, T, F, (C, D, G) | K, R, Y (A) [H, F][d] |
| A*1101 | L, M, I, V, S, A, T, G, N, (C, D, F) | K, (R) [H], Y[c] |
| A*2401 | Y, F (M) [W] | F, L, I, W [M] |
| Allele | Position 3 | Position 9 or 10 |
| A*0101 | D, E (A, S) | Y |

[a]Aminoacids are considered preferred residues when the binding of polyalanine analogues bearing such residues in the anchor position to the respective HLA-A allele is within tenfold of the parental peptide

[b]Aminoacids in parentheses are residues that are tolerated—that is, analogues carrying these substitutions bind, but less strongly (10- to 100-fold decrease in binding affinity)

[c]A T at position 9 or 10 for A*0201 and a Y for A*1101 are added as anchor residues based on the analysis of Kast *et al* (1944) and Kubo *et al* (1994)

[d]Aminoacids in brackets are thought to bind based on chemical similarity

## EFFICIENCY OF MOTIFS IN IDENTIFYING MHC BINDING PEPTIDES

We have measured the binding affinity for five HLA-A alleles: HLA-A*0101, A*0201, A*0301, A*1101 and A*2401 of an unbiased set of all possible nonamer peptides (n=240) of human papillomavirus type 16 E6 and E7 proteins. High affinity binding peptides were identified for each of the alleles. Thus, this unbiased set of peptides allowed an evaluation of the predictive value of HLA motifs derived either from the analysis of sequencing of pools of naturally processed peptides or from the binding analysis of polyalanine nonameric peptides that differed in the aminoacids present at the anchor positions. The data from this analysis are summarized in Table 4. Whereas pool sequencing derived motifs were present in only 27% of high affinity binders, the more expanded motif, based on analysis of different aminoacid substitutions at the an-

**TABLE 4. Fractions of peptides carrying HLA-A*0101, A*0201, A*0301, A*1101 or A*2401 motifs**

| Binding affinity | Pool sequencing motif | | Expanded motif | |
|---|---|---|---|---|
| High binders | 6/22 | (27%) | 20/22 | (91%) |
| Weak binders | 3/17 | (18%) | 7/17 | (41%) |
| Non-binders | 5/1161 | (0.5%) | 84/1161 | (7%) |
| Total | 14 | | 111 | |

Fractions in this table were obtained by combining all peptide/HLA binding instances for the five different alleles considered

**TABLE 5. A*0201 binding of peptides of viral and tumour origin containing canonical 2/9 anchors**

| Source | Peptide sequence | | | | | | | | | 50% inhibitory dose (nM) |
|---|---|---|---|---|---|---|---|---|---|---|
| HBV | W | **L** | S | L | L | V | P | F | **V** | 6.9 |
| HCV | Y | **L** | V | A | Y | Q | A | T | **V** | 45 |
| HBV | S | **L** | Y | A | V | S | P | S | **V** | 64 |
| *c-erb2* | H | **L** | Y | Q | G | C | Q | V | **V** | 147 |
| HIV | L | **L** | W | K | G | E | G | A | **V** | 217 |
| p53 | L | **L** | G | R | N | S | F | E | **V** | 357 |
| HCV | Y | **L** | V | T | R | H | A | D | **V** | 454 |
| HIV | I | **L** | K | E | P | V | H | G | **V** | 909 |
| HCV | G | **L** | R | D | L | A | V | A | **V** | 1 470 |
| *c-erb2* | P | **L** | T | S | I | I | S | A | **V** | 3 333 |
| HIV | H | **L** | E | G | K | V | I | L | **V** | 8 333 |
| HBV | H | **L** | S | L | R | G | L | P | **V** | 12 500 |
| HPV | R | **L** | C | V | Q | S | T | H | **V** | 16 666 |
| HPV | E | **L** | R | H | Y | S | D | S | **V** | –[1] |
| *c-erb2* | D | **L** | A | A | R | N | V | L | **V** | – |
| *c-erb2* | V | **L** | V | K | S | P | N | H | **V** | – |
| HIV | E | **L** | H | P | D | K | W | T | **V** | – |
| HBV | C | **L** | T | F | G | R | E | T | **V** | – |

9-mer peptides containing the $L_2V_9$ anchors were selected from viral or tumour protein sequences and tested for A*0201 binding. The binding is expressed as the nanomolar dose of peptide that yielded 50% inhibition of the standard peptide. A dash indicates an inhibitory dose of >50 000 nM

HBV = Hepatitis B virus; HCV = hepatitis C virus; HIV = human immunodeficiency virus; HPV = human papillomavirus

chor positions, was present in 91% of high affinity binders. Thus, the extended motifs identify the great majority, but not all, of the possible peptides capable of binding a particular allele, confirming the importance of motifs in defining MHC binding peptides.

## THE ROLE OF SECONDARY ANCHOR RESIDUES IN DETERMINING PEPTIDE BINDING TO MHC

To probe the role of positions other than the 2,9 anchor positions, a selection of 18 peptides of various viral origins, all sharing the $L_2V_9$ HLA-A*0201 motif, were synthesized and tested for A*0201 binding (Table 5). It was found that despite the presence of identical main anchor residues, the binding affinity varied in this set of naturally occurring peptide sequences over a 10 000-fold range, from 7 nmol to greater than 50 μmol. To expand this analysis, a larger library of motif containing peptides was generated. The sequences of various viral and tumour antigens were scanned for the presence of 9-mer and 10-mer peptides containing canonical 2/9 or 2/10 A*0201 motifs, as defined above. By this approach, a total of 161 9-mer peptides and 170 10-mer peptides contain-

**TABLE 6. A*0201 binding capacity of motif containing 9-mer peptides**

| Binding capacity (kDa) | Number of 9-mers |
|---|---|
| Good (≤ 50 nM) | 19 (11.8%) |
| Intermediate (50–500 nM) | 36 (22.4%) |
| Weak (500 nM–50 μM | 58 (36%) |
| Negative (> 50 μM) | 48 (29.8%) |
| Total | 161 (100%) |

Peptides containing the canonical anchors L or M in position 2 and V, L or I in the C-terminus were selected from protein sequences of viral or tumour origin, synthesized and tested for A*0201 binding, and the 50% inhibitory concentration was calculated. Peptides were separated according to their binding capacity into the indicated groups. The numbers of peptides belonging to each group and their percentage of the total number of peptides tested are given

ing an L or M in position 2 and a V, I or L in the C-terminal position were selected, synthesized and tested for binding to HLA-A*0201 molecules.

In good agreement with the data shown in Table 5, large variations in A*0201 binding affinity were detected. More specifically, as shown in Table 6, only 11.8% of the 9-mer peptides were high affinity binders ($k_D$, <50 nmol), and 22.4% of the peptides bound with intermediate affinity ($k_D$, 50–500 nmol), 36% were weak binders ($k_D$, 0.5–50 nmol) and 29.8% had no detectable binding ($k_D$, >50 μmol). It should be noted that the choice of the different binding categories used in this study was derived from two sets of experimental observations. Firstly, 80% of the known HLA restricted epitopes examined so far bind in the high affinity category, with a $k_D$ of <50 nmol, with 20% in the "intermediate" category (50–500 nmol). Secondly, 90% of MHC bound naturally processed peptides tested so far bind with a $k_D$ of <50 nmol, with 10% in the 50–500 nmol range (unpublished data). Thus, the available data indicate that good and intermediate binders are associated with functional activity.

To define more specifically what factors other than size and major anchor residues are important for A*0201 binding capacity, the following analysis was performed (Ruppert *et al*, 1993). We reasoned that aminoacid residues that facilitated high affinity binding would be overrepresented in high affinity peptides, whereas aminoacid residues that were detrimental to high affinity binding would be underrepresented in high affinity binders and overrepresented in non-binders. Accordingly, we calculated the frequency of each aminoacid in each of the non-anchor positions for the 55 high and intermediate affinity binders and the 48 non-binders found in the 9-mer peptide set. Aminoacids of similar characteristics were grouped together to increase the number of data points in each category. An example of this analysis for position 3 in the 9-mer peptide set is shown in Table 7. Several striking trends were revealed. For example, the frequency of aromatic residues (Y, F and W) was greatly increased in binding but not in non-binding peptides (21.8% v. 4.2%). Conversely, whereas 12.5% of the non-binders carried a negative charge (D or E) at posi-

**TABLE 7. Frequency of various aminoacid groups in position 3 of 9-mer peptides**

| Aminoacid group | Number of peptides (%) Good and intermediate binders | | Non-binders | | Ratio |
|---|---|---|---|---|---|
| A | 2 | (3.6) | 2 | (3.6) | 0.9 |
| G | 2 | (3.6) | 4 | (8.3) | 0.4 |
| D,E | 0 | (0) | 6 | (12.5) | 0.0 |
| R,H,K | 2 | (3.6) | 8 | (16.7) | 0.2 |
| L,V,I,M | 19 | (34.5) | 9 | (18.8) | 1.8 |
| Y,F,W | 12 | (21.8) | 2 | (4.2) | 5.2 |
| Q,N | 3 | (5.5) | 7 | (14.6) | 0.4 |
| S,T,C | 11 | (20) | 5 | (10.4) | 1.9 |
| P | 4 | (7.3) | 5 | (10.4) | 0.7 |
| Total | 55 | (100) | 48 | (100) | |

An example is given for the calculation of ratios to determine the association of certain residues with good or poor binding. Altogether, 161 9-mer peptides containing the canonical anchors L or M in position 2 and V, L or I in position 9 were selected from protein sequences of viral or tumour origin, synthesized and tested for A°0201 binding. From this set, the 55 good and intermediate binders, as well as the 48 peptides with no detectable binding, were compared in this analysis. The number of peptides in these two groups that contained a certain residue in position 3 and the frequency of occurrence of a certain residue are given. From the values obtained for the two groups a ratio was calculated for each residue or group of residues to indicate whether a residue occurs preferentially in good/intermediate binders (ratio >1) or non-binders (ratio <1)

tion 3, these same residues were completely absent at this position in the subset of high and intermediate A°0201 binding peptides. Similarly, positively charged residues (R, K and H) were much more frequent in non-binders than

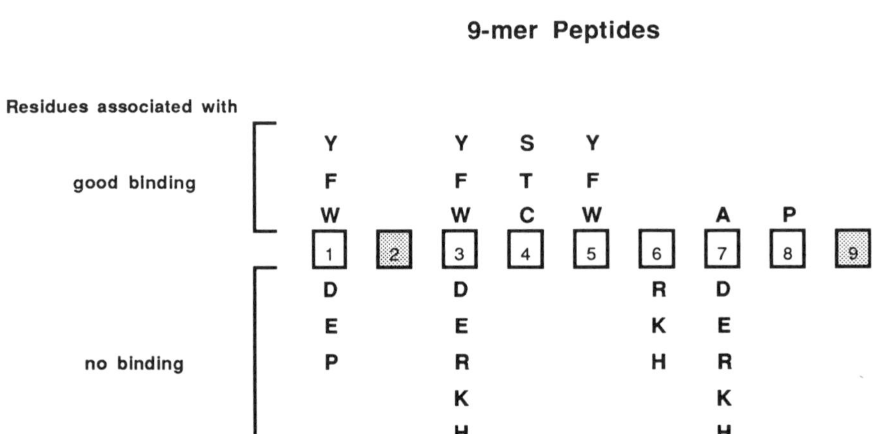


**Fig. 2.** Summary of secondary effects in HLA-A*0201 binding. Residues strongly associated with good or poor A*0201 binding. Based on the ratios described in Table 6, residues are shown that were found to be associated with good binding (ratio >4) or poor binding (ratio <0.25) in a given position in 9-mer peptides. Anchor residues in all peptides were L or M in position 2, and L, V or I in the C-terminal position

in binders (16.7% v. 3.6%). To quantitate these differences more conveniently, the frequency of a given aminoacid group in A°0201 binders was divided by the frequency in non-binders to obtain a "frequency ratio". This ratio indicates whether a given group of residues occurs at a given position preferentially in binders (ratio >1) or in non-binders (ratio <1).

To facilitate analysis of the data, a threshold level was set for the ratios, such that residues that had a greater frequency of more than fourfold in binders than in non-binders were regarded as favoured or preferred residues, and residues that had a lower frequency of more than fourfold in binders than in non-binders were regarded as unfavoured or deleterious residues. Following this approach, groups of residues showing prominent associations with either A°0201 binding capacity or lack thereof were identified. A summary of this analysis for all positions other than 2 and 9 is shown in Fig. 2. In general, the most detrimental effects were observed with charged aminoacids. At position 1, both P and acid residues were infrequent in A°0201 binding peptides. At position 6, base residues were associated with non-binding peptides, whereas both acid and base residues were infrequent in good binders at pos-

**TABLE 8. Validation of the extended motifs using an independent set of 9-mer peptides**

| Source | Position | Sequence | | | | | | | | | 50% dose (nM) |
|---|---|---|---|---|---|---|---|---|---|---|---|
| *Peptides carrying no deleterious residues:* | | | | | | | | | | | |
| HBV | 1406 | S | L | **Y** | A | D | S | P | S | V | 14 |
| HBV | 204 | **F** | L | G | G | T | T | V | C | L | 29 |
| HBV | 1286 | **F** | L | C | K | Q | Y | L | N | L | 29 |
| HBV | 1045 | G | L | S | R | **Y** | V | A | R | L | 42 |
| HIV | 280 | R | M | **Y** | **S** | P | I | S | I | L | 56 |
| MAGE | 101 | A | L | S | R | K | V | **A** | E | L | 100 |
| *Peptides carrying deleterious residues:* | | | | | | | | | | | |
| HBV | 1154 | H | L | *E* | **S** | L | F | T | A | V | 10 000 |
| HBV | 1052 | R | L | S | **S** | N | S | *R* | I | L | 10 000 |
| HBV | 1420 | *D* | L | V | H | **F** | A | S | P | L | 16 667 |
| PAP | 201 | *D* | L | **F** | G | I | W | S | K | V | 25 000 |
| MAGE | 147 | S | L | *R* | V | L | A | A | G | L | – |
| HBV | 511 | N | M | G | L | K | F | *R* | Q | L | – |
| HBV | 83 | *D* | L | V | V | S | Y | V | N | V | – |
| MAGE | 143 | *D* | L | Q | Q | S | L | *R* | V | L | – |
| PAP | 352 | *P* | L | *E* | R | **F** | A | *E* | L | V | – |

Two independent sets of 9-mer peptides not previously analysed were studied for binding. The 50% inhibitory dose of these peptides represents the average of at least two independent experiments. A dash indicates a 50% dose of greater than 50 000 nM. Peptides were sorted by whether or not they contained a deleterious residue. Residues associated with poor binding, as listed in Fig. 2, are italicized underlined and residues associated with good binding are shown in bold.

MAGE = Melanoma associated gene expression antigen; PAP = prostatic acid phosphatase

**TABLE 9. Correlation of A*0201 binding and the presence or absence of preferred or deleterious residues**

| Residues in non-anchor positions | | Binders | Weak and non-binders | |
|---|---|---|---|---|
| preferred | detrimental | ($k_D \le 500$ nM) | ($k_D > 500$ nM–50 μM) | Total |
| ≥ 1 | 0 | 83 | 38 | 121 |
| 0 or ≥ 1 | ≥ 1 | 19 | 208 | 227 |
| Total | | 102 | 246 | 348 |

All peptides listed in this study containing canonical anchors in position 2 and the C-terminus were grouped according to the presence of preferred residues or deleterious residues (with or without the presence of preferred residues) as defined in Fig. 2 and according to their binding capacity, as indicated

itions 3 and 7. Conversely, aromatic residues were associated with high affinity binding at positions 1, 3 and 5. Furthermore, residues with OH or SH contain ing side chains S, T or C were favoured at position 4, whereas A was favoured at position 7 and P in position 8.

The value of the above analysis for predicting HLA-A*0201 binding was examined using independent panels of 9-mer peptides (Table 8). For this purpose, the following two sets were synthesized: six peptides that contained no unfavoured residues and at least one favoured residue, and a set of nine peptides that carried at least one unfavoured residue in their sequence. All peptides contained canonical anchor residues at position 2 (L or M) and position 9 (L, V or I). When their binding capacity was determined, it was found that four of six peptides carrying no unfavoured residues and one or more favoured residues bound with high affinity (<50 nmol), and the remaining two bound in the 50–100 nmol range. By contrast, none of the peptides carrying an unfavoured residue bound HLA-A*0201 with high affinity, with only four peptides demonstrating any detectable binding in the 10–25 μmol range. Interestingly, peptides carrying both one favoured residue and one or more unfavoured residues were found to be poor or negative binders.

A compilation of all the data available for this kind of analysis is shown in Table 9. A total of 348 peptides, all carrying canonical anchor residues in positions 2 and 9, have been tested for A*0201 binding. Peptides were divided into two groups: (a) no detrimental residues, and one or more favoured residues, and (b) one or more detrimental residues. The frequencies of good and intermediate binders ($k_D$, <500 nmol), weak binders ($k_D$, 0.5–50 μmol) and non-binders in each peptide group are shown in Table 9. Of the 121 peptides that contained no unfavoured and at least one favoured residue(s), 83 (69%) were good or intermediate binders. By contrast, of the 227 peptides carrying one or more unfavoured residues, only 19 (8%) bound A*0201 with high or intermediate affinity. Thus, the value of this expanded motif for predicting high and intermediate binding peptides of 69% is more than twice that of the 29% (102 of 348) found when these peptides were analysed only on the basis of containing the canonical 2/9 anchor motif.

**TABLE 10. Only high or intermediate affinity peptides are immunogenic**

| Peptide | | | | | | | | | Binding ICM (μM) | Immunogenicity | |
|---|---|---|---|---|---|---|---|---|---|---|---|
| | | | | | | | | | | 1 nM | 50 nM |
| F | **L** | L | S | L | G | I | H | **L** | .107 | + | + |
| G | **L** | Y | S | S | T | V | P | **V** | .370 | – | + |
| H | **L** | Y | S | H | P | I | I | **L** | .430 | – | + |
| W | **L** | L | R | G | T | S | F | **V** | 3.1 | – | – |
| N | **L** | S | W | L | S | L | D | **V** | 4.3 | – | – |
| L | **L** | S | S | N | L | S | W | **L** | 12.1 | – | – |
| N | **L** | O | S | L | T | N | L | **L** | 22.4 | – | – |
| H | **L** | L | V | G | S | S | G | **L** | 31.0 | – | – |
| L | **L** | D | D | E | A | G | P | **L** | 280.0 | – | – |
| P | **L** | E | E | E | L | P | R | **L** | 560.0 | – | – |
| D | **L** | N | L | G | N | L | N | **V** | – | – | – |
| N | **L** | Y | V | S | L | L | L | **L** | – | – | – |
| P | **L** | P | I | H | T | A | E | **L** | – | – | – |

HLA-A°0201 $K^b$ transgenic mice (Vitiello *et al,* 1991) were immunized subcutaneously in incomplete Freund's adjuvant with 1 nM or 50 nM of the indicated peptides, plus 50 nM of the T helper epitope. Spleen cells were tested for peptide specific/HLA-A°0201 restricted cytotoxic T lymphocyte activity, as previously described (Vitiello *et al,* 1991)

## BINDING AFFINITY FOR MHC AND IMMUNOGENICITY

As described above, the great majority of previously defined T cell epitopes, when tested for binding to their respective HLA restriction elements, demonstrate high affinity binding, and the remainder show intermediate binding affinity for the restriction element. This suggests that high (<50 nmol) and intermediate (50–500 nmol) affinity defines the affinity of interaction with MHC required to induce an immune response. To further explore the relationship between antigenicity and MHC binding affinity, a series of HLA-A2 binding peptides with varying affinities were used to immunize HLA-A2 transgenic mice. The results, shown in Table 10, indicate that only peptides with high and intermediate affinity for MHC were immunogenic, with $k_D$ values varying between 100 and 500 nmol. Furthermore, when the immunizing dose was decreased, only the highest affinity peptide was immunogenic. These data further substantiate the importance of MHC binding affinity in determining the immunogenicity of motif containing peptides.

## SUMMARY

In this chapter, we have defined the structural motifs that dictate the capacity of peptides to bind to five different HLA-A alleles that represent some of the most common alleles found in different ethnic populations. In general, these peptide motifs were very specific for the individual HLA-A alleles, with the exception of HLA-A*0301 and HLA-A*1101, for which the motifs were very similar. When these motifs were tested against an unbiased and complete set of nonamer peptides derived from human papillomavirus E6 and E7 proteins, it was found that the vast majority of high and intermediate binding peptides contained the appropriate motif. Furthermore, using the dominant anchor residues, together with the aminoacid positions that interact with secondary anchor residues, it was possible to predict high and intermediate binders. Finally, the finding that there is a direct correlation between binding affinity for MHC and immunogenicity suggests a practical application of being able to predict those peptides that have a high affinity binding for a particular MHC allele—that is, in the design of peptide based vaccines for prophylactic or therapeutic use.

## References

Bjorkman PJ, Saper MA, Samraoui B, Bennett SW, Strominger JL and Wiley DC (1987) Structure of the human class I histocompatibility antigen, HLA-A2. *Nature* **329** 506–512

Central Data Analysis Committee (1992) Allele frequencies, Section 6.3: Splits Combined (Five Loci), In: Tsuji K, Aizawa M and Sasazuki T (eds). *The Proceedings of the Eleventh International Histocompatibility Workshop and Conference,* held in Yokohama, Japan, 6–13 November 1991, pp 1066–1077, Oxford University Press, Tokyo

Cerundolo V, Elliott T, Elvin J, Bastin J, Rammensee H-G and Townsend A (1991) The binding affinity and dissociation rates of peptides for class I major histocompatibility complex molecules. *European Journal of Immunology* **21** 2069–2075

Falk K, Rötzschke O, Stevanovic S, Jung G and Rammensee HG (1991) Allele-specific motifs revealed by sequencing of self-peptides eluted from MHC molecules. *Nature* **351** 290–296

Fremont DH, Matsumura M, Stura EA, Peterson PA and Wilson IA (1992) Crystal structures of two viral peptides in complex with murine MHC class I H-2K$^b$. *Science* **257** 919–927

Jardetzky TS, Gorga JC, Busch R, Rothbard J, Strominger JL and Wiley DC (1990) Peptide binding to HLA-DR1: a peptide with most residues substituted to alanine retains MHC binding. *EMBO Journal* **9** 1797–1803

Kast WM, Brandt RMP, Sidney J *et al* (1994) The role of HLA-A motifs in identification of potential CTL epitopes in human papillomavirus type 16 E6 and E7 proteins. *Journal of Immunology* **152:** 3904–3912

Kubo RT, Sette A, Grey HM *et al* (1994) Definition of specific peptide motifs for four major HLA-A alleles. *Journal of Immunology* **152:** 3913–3924

Rötzschke O, Falk K, Deres K *et al* (1990) Isolation and analysis of naturally processed viral peptides as recognized by cytotoxic T cells. *Nature* **348** 252–254

Ruppert J, Sidney J, Celis E, Kubo RT, Grey HM and Sette A (1993) Prominent role of secondary anchors in peptide binding to HLA-A*0201 molecules. *Cell* **74** 929–937

Saper MA, Bjorkman PJ and Wiley DC (1991) Refined structure of the human histocompatibility antigen HLA-A2 at 2.6Å resolution. *Journal of Molecular Biology* **219** 277–319

Sette A, O'Sullivan D, Krieger JI, Karr RW, Lamont AG and Grey HM (1991) MHC-antigen-T cell interactions: an overview, In: Gefter ML (ed). *Seminars in Immunology,* vol 3, pp 195–202, Saunders, Philadelphia

Sette, A, Southwood S, O'Sullivan D, Gaeta FCA, Sidney J and Grey HM (1992) Effect of pH on class II-peptide interactions. *Journal of Immunology* **148** 844–851

Van Bleek GM and Nathenson SG (1990) Isolation of an endogenously processed immunodominant viral peptide from the class I H-2K$^b$ molecule. *Nature* **348** 213–216

Vitiello A, Marchesini D, Furze J, Sherman LA and Chesnut RW (1991) Analysis of the HLA-restricted influenza-specific cytotoxic T lymphocyte response in transgenic mice carrying a chimeric human-mouse class I major histocompatibility complex. *Journal of Experimental Medicine* **173** 1007–1015

The authors are responsible for the accuracy of the references.

# Recognition of Viral Antigens at the Cell Surface

**ANDREW MCMICHAEL • PAUL KLENERMAN**
**SARAH ROWLAND-JONES • FRANCES GOTCH • PAUL MOSS**
*Institute of Molecular Medicine, John Radcliffe Hospital, Oxford*



## INTRODUCTION

It is a pleasure to contribute to this volume in honour of Mike Crumpton. Our scientific paths have crossed on several occasions in the past 20 years. In the context of this review, we collaborated on experiments investigating HLA-A2 variants detected by cytotoxic T lymphocytes (CTL) (Gotch *et al,* 1985), and we worked together on the MRC AIDS Directed Programme Steering Committee. This last interaction gives me the opportunity to discuss recognition of HIV by cytotoxic T lymphocytes in the role of these cells in control of this infection. In the past 7 years, the function of class I major histocompatibility complex (MHC) molecules in presenting antigen has been defined. Zinkernagel and Doherty (1974, 1979) had shown, in 1974, that CTL recognized viral antigens at the surface of infected cells in association with class I MHC molecules. The results of the experiments suggested either that there were two receptors, one for MHC and one for virus, or that the T cell receptor recognized a complex of virus antigen and MHC antigen. When it was shown that T lymphocytes, including CTL, carried a single receptor that conferred both specificities on transfection (Dembic *et al,* 1986), it was obvious that the latter hypothesis was correct. Meanwhile, Townsend and colleagues (1985, 1986) had shown that influenza specific CTL could recognize fragments of internal viral protein, such as the nucleoprotein, transfected into target cells. They also demonstrated that CTL recognized peptide fragments of nucleoprotein presented by class I MHC molecules and that different MHC molecules presented different peptides (McMichael *et al,* 1986; Townsend *et al,* 1986). The crystal structure of HLA-A2 (Bjorkman *et al,* 1987a,b) revealed a peptide binding site within the MHC molecule, in a groove on the membrane-distal surface. In the original crystal, this groove contained unresolvable electron density, which was suggested to be a mixture of peptides (Bjorkman *et al,* 1987a,b). Direct evidence for this came from experiments by Rammensee (Falk *et al,* 1990; Rotzschke and Falk, 1991) and Van Bleek and Nathenson (1990), who eluted peptides from purified class I molecules. Subsequently, class I molecules were crystallized with single peptides (Fremont, 1992; Guo *et al,* 1992; Zhang *et al,* 1992), formally proving that the groove does indeed bind peptides.

Recent experiments have revealed how peptides reach the MHC groove (Townsend and Trowsdale, 1993). Cytoplasmic proteins are degraded by proteases in the cytosol, most probably by the proteasome complex (Goldberg and Rock, 1992; Michalek *et al,* 1993). The peptides generated are transported by the transporters TAP1 and TAP2, both encoded in the class II region of the MHC, into the endoplasmic reticulum (Townsend and Trowsdale, 1993). Here, peptides of the optimal length (8 to 12 aminoacids) bind to the groove of the nascent heavy chain (Elliott *et al,* 1992) or to the newly formed heavy chain $\beta_2$ microglobulin complex (Townsend *et al,* 1990).

## BINDING OF PEPTIDES TO MHC CLASS I MOLECULES

Analysis of the peptides eluted from class I molecules shows that they are most commonly 9 aminoacids long but sometimes 8, 10, 11 or 12 residues long. Crystallographic analysis of bound peptides shows that they bind in the grooves of the class I molecules as extended chains with the N-terminus and C-terminus fitting into conserved pockets at either end of the groove. The invariant aminoacids in these MHC pockets include tyrosines and threonines that hydrogen bond to the termini. The same bonding patterns are formed at the termini of the peptides whatever their length, the difference being the degree of arching of the peptide out of the groove (Guo *et al,* 1992). Falk and colleagues (1991) sequenced the peptide mixtures eluted from class I MHC molecules and found that, for any given class I molecule, there were conserved aminoacids at particular residues. For instance, peptides that bind to HLA-A2 have a leucine or isoleucine at position 2, H-2D$^b$ binding peptides have a tyrosine at position 5 and there is an arginine at position 2 in peptides that bind to HLA-B27. In addition, the C-terminal aminoacids are conserved. These conserved residues are termed anchors, and it has been argued that their side chains would fit into pockets that are characteristic of the particular class I molecule. Crystallographic studies have shown this to be correct. Thus, it is possible to identify aminoacid sequence motifs characteristic for class I MHC molecule, and those so identified are shown in Table 1. These motifs can be defined by comparing eluted peptides or peptide epitopes that have been optimized to the length that binds most efficiently, either sensitizing

**TABLE 1. Sequence motifs of peptides binding to class I MHC molecules**

| | Aminoacid at residues | | | | | | |
|---|---|---|---|---|---|---|---|
| MHC | 1 | 2 | 3 | 4 | 5 | -------- | C′ |
| H-2D$^b$ | | | | | N | | M/I |
| H-2K$^b$ | | | | | F/Y | | L/I |
| H-2K$^d$ | | Y | | | | | L/I |
| H-2K$^k$ | | E/D | | | | | I |
| H-2L$^d$ | | P | | | | | L |
| HLA-A1 | | | | | | | |
| HLA-A2 | | L | | | | | V/L |
| HLA-A3.1 | | I/L | F | | | | K/Y |
| HLA-A11 | | I/L | | | | | K |
| HLA-A68 | | T/V | | | | | R |
| HLA-B7 | A | P | R | | | | L/V |
| HLA-B8 | | | K/R | | K/R | | I/L |
| HLA-B27 | | R | | | | | K/R |
| HLA-B35 | | P | | | | | Y |
| HLA-B53 | | P | | | | | F/W |

target cells for lysis at the lowest concentration or binding at the lowest concentration. Although there are exceptions to these motifs, they are particularly useful in identifying peptide epitopes within sequences. Candidate epitopes can be checked for binding to the MHC molecules and then tested with CTL (eg Hill *et al,* 1992). Not all peptides that bind are epitopes, but all proven epitopes bind in these assays.

The aminoacid at the C-terminus is always an anchor. Furthermore, there is great restriction in the aminoacids at this position (Elliott *et al,* 1993). The commonest residues used are isoleucine, leucine, valine, tyrosine, arginine and lysine. These residues appear to fit the structure of the F pocket within the groove centred above residue 116 in the floor of the MHC class I molecule (Elliott *et al,* 1993). On the side of this pocket, residue 77 also appears to be important. Thus, if 116 and 77 are aspartic acids, the C-terminal residue of the peptide is most commonly arginine or lysine, if 116 is tyrosine, the C-terminal aminoacid is isoleucine, leucine or valine, if 116 is serine, the C-terminus of the peptide is commonly tyrosine. The restricted aminoacids at the C-terminus fit well with the hypothesis that the peptides are generated from cytoplasmic proteins by the proteasome complex. This cleaves at the carboxy side of hydrophobic, positively charged and negatively charged aminoacids. These enzymes could therefore provide peptides with the "correct" C-termini. The exceptions are the negatively charged C-termini, which have so far not been identified in any peptides bound to any class I molecule. Two components of the proteasome complex, LMP2 and LMP7, encoded within the MHC, may restrict the enzymatic activity of cleaving at the carboxy side of acidic aminoacids (Djaballah and Rivett, 1992; Driscoll *et al,* 1993). The transporters may also select for the C-terminus of aminoacids, again fitting with the C-terminus preferred by the class I molecules (Neefjes *et al,* 1993; Shepherd *et al,* 1993). There are no such restrictions at the N-terminus, and it is likely that the final peptide bound in the groove is cleaved at the N-terminus by different enzymes. There is some evidence that longer peptides are trimmed in the lumen of the endoplasmic reticulum. This might happen with the peptide floating free or with the peptide partially bound to the MHC complex (Rotzschke and Falk, 1991).

These processes are not limited to virally encoded proteins. There are abundant self protein peptides within the class I molecules at the surface of any cell. It has been shown that the HLA-A2 molecules on a B lymphoblastoid cell line may contain more than 1000 different peptides (Hunt *et al,* 1992). Probably fewer than five of these are derived from Epstein-Barr virus, the transforming virus. Virally derived proteins will elicit immune responses because they are foreign and T cells have the potential to react with them but will only do this provided they obtain a threshold of at least 100 peptide molecules per cell (Christinck *et al,* 1991). Virally derived peptides must compete within the endoplasmic reticulum with self derived peptides and, to get above this threshold, they will either have to bind with high affinity or be expressed in great excess.

## CYTOTOXIC T LYMPHOCYTES IN HIV INFECTION

Human immunodeficiency virus (HIV), the AIDS virus, is a retrovirus with a well characterized infectious cycle (Peterlin and Luciw, 1988). The virus binds by the interaction of gp120 with CD4 (Dalgleish *et al,* 1984) and enters cells, and viral RNA is then reverse transcribed to cDNA. The latter is integrated, in activated T cells or macrophages, into the genome, where it may remain latent or continue the activation process and express mRNA and viral RNA to generate new viral particles that bud from the infected cell. Susceptibility to CTL attack comes during the second part of this cycle with the expression of viral proteins before release of viral particles. Insufficient viral protein is taken into cells on infection to generate epitopes before viral protein synthesis (Nixon DF and McMichael AJ, unpublished).

Human immunodeficiency virus specific CTL are surprisingly easy to demonstrate in patients infected with HIV (Plata *et al,* 1987; Walker *et al,* 1987; Nixon *et al,* 1988). They have been demonstrated, as shown in Fig. 1, at the time of clearance of the initial viraemia before the appearance of neutralizing antibody (Koup R *et al,* personnal communication). During the subsequent phase of the infection, when the patient is still symptom free, CTL activity can be extremely high and demonstrable in peripheral blood lymphocytes without any culture in vitro (Plata *et al,* 1987; Walker *et al,* 1987). Over several years, this CTL activity declines slightly but remains detectable until quite late, whereas the CD4 count gradually declines and virus replicates at a low level.

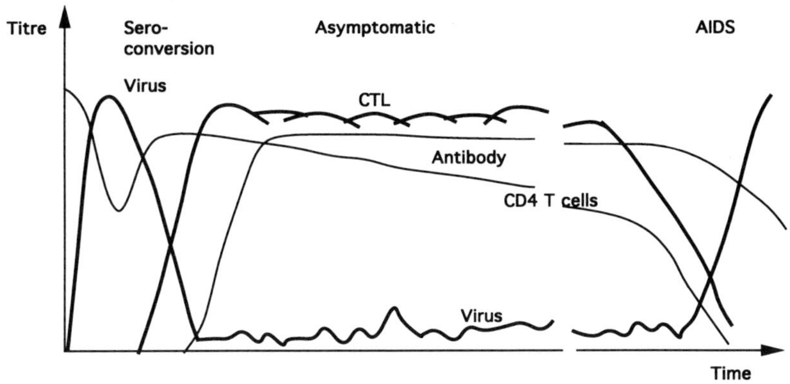


**Fig. 1.** The immune response to HIV. The schematic view shows the viraemia, CTL activity, antibody level and CD4 count for a period of (usually) years following infection with HIV

During this phase, however, there is widespread virus infection, particularly in lymph nodes, where up to 25% of CD4 T cells may be infected (Embretson *et al,* 1993; Pantaleo *et al,* 1993). After a variable period, usually several years, AIDS develops. In patients with full blown AIDS, HIV specific CTL activity is normally undetectable. There is a period preceding this when CD4 counts drop, sometimes precipitously, and CTL activity may be present or absent or may fluctuate. There is a documented decline in CTL activity around the time of the onset of AIDS (Hoffenbach *et al,* 1989; Carmichael *et al,* 1993).

In the initial phase of HIV infection, the pattern of CTL activity is reminiscent of other acute and chronic virus infections. The CTL may well be responsible for the initial clearance of the viraemia. In other persistent virus infections, CTL activity remains moderately high and is thought to control the virus infection indefinitely. What goes wrong in HIV infection?

We have identified two problems in HIV infection that may contribute to the ultimate failure of the CTL response to control the infection. The first is the overstimulation of CTL activity, which could lead to T cell clonal exhaustion, and in the presence of declining CD4 (helper Th1) T cell activity could lead to failure of new CTL responses to replace those that are exhausted. The second problem results from virus variability, which frequently affects epitope binding to MHC or presentation to T cells. Comparison of all the isolates of HIV indicates considerable variability in all proteins, particularly the virus envelope (Holmes *et al,* 1992). The latter is thought to be selected by the antibody response and is somewhat similar to variability occurring in influenza haemagglutinin, although in the case of HIV, the variability also occurs within single patients. Diversity is also found in the internal proteins, such as gag, pol and nef, which make the major CTL epitope donors (Myers *et al,* 1992). Analysis of the variability in the isolates of HIV1 gag reveals that every part of the protein can vary and that there is no conserved nine aminoacid stretch that does not have some variability. Thus, viral escape from CTL control is a real possibility. The variability is generated by errors in reverse transcription, coupled with the continuous replication of this virus in infected individuals. Thus, there is accumulation of mutant virus throughout the period of infection (Wain-Hobson, 1993).

## T CELL EXHAUSTION

The high level of CTL activity in HIV infected individuals is remarkable. Lysis of HIV infected targets in an HLA restricted manner by uncultured peripheral blood lymphocytes is unique to HIV and HTLVI (Jacobson *et al,* 1990). The level of lysis seen in these fresh CTL lytic assays implies very high levels of circulating effector CTL. For instance, in one patient we have studied, we regularly see 30% lysis at an effector:target ratio of 30 peripheral blood lymphocytes to 1 target cell. The same level of lysis can be achieved by CTL clones at around 0.25:1 (Rowland-Jones S, unpublished). This implies that CTL are present at around 1% of peripheral blood lymphocytes. Experiments in which unique DNA sequence markers for the CDR3 region of the Vβ chain of the dominant CTL clones recognizing particular peptide-MHC complexes in this and two other patients indicate that the dominant clones may represent about 1% of peripheral blood lymphocytes (Moss P, Rowland-Jones S, Frodsham P, McMichael A and Bell J, unpublished). This experiment was done by amplifying T cell receptor, cDNA from peripheral blood lymphocytes of patients by means of an anchor polymerase chain reaction technique cloning the positives into bacteriophage M13, transforming *Escherichia coli* and then probing with TCR and CDR3 specific probes. Exact conservation of CDR3 was confirmed by sequencing. Repeated experiments, probing thousands of clones, gave the figure of 1%. However, when a standard limiting dilution assay (LDA) was carried out in the same patients, the level of CTL precursor cells was much lower (Gotch *et al,* 1990). In the LDA, peripheral blood lymphocytes are seeded at low numbers into microtitre wells, then cultured with peptide epitope, feeder cells and optimal cytokines, and lytic activity is measured after 10–14 days. This assay allows precursor clones to grow up to a level where they can be detected in CTL assays. The LDA is thought to give an accurate measure of the number of precursors present in the peripheral blood, and in these patients, it gave levels of 1 in 5000 to 1 in 10 000. These frequencies are a little higher than those seen for precursors for Epstein-Barr virus specific CTL.

There is clearly a discrepancy between the figures of 1% for active CTL and 0.05% for memory CTL. Two possibilities should be considered. Firstly, there could be some form of suppression of CTL growth so that the number of CTL presursors is underestimated; Joly and colleagues (1989) have reported that CTL responses may be suppressed in HIV infected patients, but this needs further investigation. The second mechanism might be through terminal differentiation of overstimulated CTL (Gotch *et al,* 1990), a process that has been found in a mouse model (Moskaphidis *et al,* 1993). If this is the case, it could be possible to deplete the memory CTL population while maintaining a high level of circulating end stage effector CTL, a situation that may eventually lead to the collapse of the CTL response. We have observed one patient in whom the dominant CTL clone had almost disappeared from the blood at the time when the whole immune response to the HIV pol protein disappeared (Rowland-Jones S, Moss P, McAdam S, Bell J and McMichael A, unpublished). We believe that this could be an example of the terminal exhaustion of a dominant CTL clone and hence the response to a particular viral protein. Carmichael *et al* (1993) have obtained similar values for CTL precursors and have demonstrated that these decline to undetectable levels as the CD4 count drops below 200/mm$^3$. Carmichael A, Borysiewicz L and Sissons JP (personal communication) have also suggested that precursors from HIV infected patients particularly need added interleukin 2 (IL2), implying that the production of endogenous IL2 by CD4 T cells might be impaired. The failure in the CD4 T cell, particularly the Th1 subset, could explain why the exhausted CTL clones are not replaced by new clones. Another reason for the failure to replace the CTL response might be HIV infection of the thymus and damage to the CD8 precursors, the double positive T cells. This needs to be further explored (McCune, 1991). A further reason might be failure of dendritic cells to initiate CTL responses late in the infection (Macatonia *et al,* 1990).

## VIRUS VARIABILITY

Although some patients make very stable CTL responses to dominant peptide epitopes that are maintained over several years, others make unstable responses. The latter is particularly apparent in patients with HLA-B8, which presents three epitopes from HIV gag. In patients studied, the response switched from one to the other in an unstable fashion (Phillips *et al,* 1991). When HIV provirus from these patients was sequenced in the epitope regions, aminoacid sequence variability was found in the epitopes presented by HLA-B8. By contrast, the sequences of the epitopes presented by HLA-B27 and HLA-A2 varied very little. When synthetic peptides were made representing the variant epitopes, it was found that the HLA-B8 restricted CTL were highly susceptible to the variation. Thus, some epitopes were seen by none of the patient's CTL lines or clones, whereas others were seen by some clones but not others. Other experiments indicate that most of these peptide sequence variants do bind to HLA-B8 but that a number of them are not recognized by most CTL clones. Some of the sequence changes involve changes of the anchor lysines to arginines at positions 3 and 5 of the peptide, these anchor residues being particularly important for binding to HLA-B8. These changes may cause the peptide to be positioned slightly differently in the groove and so affect T cell recognition. We found more variability in the epitopes presented by HLA-B8 in the HLA-B8 positive patients than in HLA-B8 negative patients who make stable CTL responses to other epitopes (Phillips *et al,* 1991). This implies that there may be some selection of viruses occurring in the B8+ individuals. We have preliminary evidence for increased frequency in one of these potential escape mutants, but measurement of frequency of virus variants in peripheral blood is difficult and can probably never be completely reliable. It is clear, however, that the variants not recognized by CTL are present at sufficiently high frequencies to be detectable by repeated polymerase chain reaction amplification and sequencing in these patients over many time points. Therefore, there is considerable potential for virus escape from CTL control, particularly if the CTL response is dominated by clones specific for a small number of epitopes. Furthermore, given that most infected cells carry only a single integrated copy of provirus, all progeny of variant cells will carry the mutant, so that escape is likely, in contrast to a situation where the variant viruses are a minority subpopulation within the products of a single infected cell. It should be emphasized that the nature of escape mutation from CTL control is likely to be far less dramatic than escape from antibody control; in the former, the selective forces may well differ at different sites, so that the overall effect may be to diversify the virus rather than select single escaping virus clones.

Jameson *et al* (1993) have demonstrated in an experimental model (not HIV) that epitope peptide sequence variants, which bind to MHC but are poorly recognized, may impair the ability of CTL to recognize the normal peptide sequence. In their experiments, CTL were exposed to cells that had been pulsed with the variant peptide and were then mixed with labelled target cells exposed to the normal sequence epitope. Recognition of the latter was impaired. We have repeated these experiments with the variant sequences found in HIV in epitopes in p17 and p24 presented by HLA-B8 and -B27 (Klenerman *et al,* 1994). Similar findings were obtained, indicating that variant sequence may impair the ability of CTL to recognize other cells infected with virus carrying the normal sequence. This inhibition was found using, as the "decoy", cells infected with recombinant vaccinia virus carrying p17 with variant sequence. Therefore, the effect is not dependent on artificially high concentrations of peptides. The mechanisms by which cells expressing variant epitope sequences could impair T cell recognition are not fully understood. Experiments have ruled out competition of peptide for the MHC moleules because cells incubated in one peptide can inhibit recognition of separate cells incubated with the natural peptide and of cells infected with vaccinia expressing the wild type sequence. It seems likely that the fault lies at the level of T cell receptor interaction with the peptide-MHC complex. If this is low affinity, a negative signal may be given to the T cells. These experiments suggest an unexpected way in which virus variation may impair the CTL response to normal virus sequence, giving further impetus to escape from CTL control.

The experiments on epitope variability and its effects imply that the nature of the CTL response in HIV infected patients is affected by the HLA type. Some HLA molecules select relatively invariant epitopes or are more permissive of epitope variation, whereas other HLA molecules may, by chance, select more variable parts of the virus or may be particularly susceptible to small sequence changes in their ability to present to T cells. Thus, HLA type should play a part in determining the effectiveness of CTL activity in HIV infection and, by implication, the survival. Three studies indicate that the HLA-B8 bearing haplotype A1 B8 DR3 is associated with poor prognosis (Steel *et al,* 1988; Kaslow *et al,* 1990; Mallal *et al,* 1990), although this was not found in another study (Mann *et al,* 1988). This may be due in part to the variability in the epitopes presented by HLA-B8, although other genes on this haplotype could well contribute to the poor prognosis. It will be worth exploring the HLA types of long term survivors and patients with rapidly progressing disease, at the extreme ends of the spectrum, to determine the extent of the HLA contribution to susceptibility.

## A MECHANISM FOR THE FAILURE OF THE IMMUNE SYSTEM TO CONTROL HIV INFECTION

If we accept a central role for CTL in controlling HIV replication (widely believed, but not yet fully proven), the following sequence of events can be proposed. Initial virus replication is controlled by the early CTL response, but virus is widely distributed in lymphoid organs by that time. The large antigenic load in CD4 positive T cells, macrophages and dendritic cells gives a strong, or overstrong, stimulus to CTL. This controls the infection but may contribute to the fall in CD4 T cells and destruction of lymphoid follicles. The response probably takes the form of waves of T cell clones; as each is exhausted, driven to terminal differentiation, new clones take their place, but these are dependent on normal thymic function and adequate help from Th1 cells. If these are impaired, then the CTL response collapses. This process is accelerated if the dominant epitopes can vary significantly in their sequence. Then the level of CTL response has to be much larger (ie involving more clones) to deal with the virus diversity. In addition, some virus epitopes may be poorly recognized by all available clones and so have some selective advantage. Escape from immune control is likely to occur earlier in these patients. A mathematical model that is consistent with this hypothesis has been proposed by Nowak *et al* (1991).

The core of this hypothesis is that CTL have a critical role in controlling HIV infection. This must be more firmly established by correlating CTL activity with control of this infection, particularly in the primate model, in which it is possible to test the role of each component of the immune system.

## SUMMARY

There is now a very good understanding of the way in which epitope peptides are generated from virus proteins and how the peptides bind to the class I

MHC molecules. This gives a framework in which to analyse the potentially protective cytotoxic T lymphocyte response in human immunodeficiency virus infection. A detailed understanding of the specificity of the responding T cells, the clonality of these T cells and the effects of virus variation on the CTL gives a possible explanation for the ultimate failure of the CTL response to control this virus infection.

## References

Bjorkman P, Saper M, Samraoui B, Bennett W, Strominger J and Wiley D (1987a) The foreign antigen binding site and T cell recognition regions of class I histocompatibility antigens. *Nature* **329** 512–519

Bjorkman P, Saper M, Samraoui B, Bennett W, Strominger J and Wiley D (1987b) Structure of human class I histocompatibility antigen, HLA-A2. *Nature* **329** 506–511

Carmichael A, Jin X, Sissons P and Borysiewicz L (1993) Quantitative analysis of the human HIV-1 specific cytotoxic T lymphocyte (CTL) response at different stages of infection: differential CTL responses to HIV-1 and Epstein-Barr virus in late disease. *Journal of Experimental Medicine* **177** 249–256

Christinck ER, Luscher MA, Barber BH and Williams DB (1991) Peptide binding to class I MHC on living cells and quantitation of complexes required for CTL lysis. *Nature* **352** 67–70

Dalgleish AG, Beverley PCL, Clapham PR, Crawford DH, Greaves MF and Weiss RA (1984) The CD4 (T4) antigen is an essential component of the receptor for the AIDS virus. *Nature* **312** 763–767

Dembic Z, Haas W, Weiss S *et al* (1986) Transfer of specificity by murine alpha and T-cell receptor genes. *Nature* **320** 232–238

Djaballah H and Rivett AJ (1992) Peptidylglutamyl-peptide hydrolase activity of the multicatalytic proteinase complex: evidence for a new high-affinity site, analysis of cooperative kinetics, and the effect of manganese ions. *Biochemistry* **31** 4133–4141

Driscoll J, Brown MG, Finlay D and Monaco JJ (1993) MHC-linked LMP gene products specifically alter peptidase activities of the proteasome. *Nature* **365** 262–264

Elliott T, Cerundolo V and Townsend A (1992) Short peptides assist the folding of free class I heavy chains in solution. *European Journal of Immunology* **22** 3121–3125

Elliott T, Driscoll P, Smith M and McMichael A J (1993) Peptide epitope selection by class I MHC molecules. *Current Biology* **3** 854–866

Embretson J, Zupancic M, Ribas JL *et al* (1993) Massive covert infection of helper T lymphocytes and macrophages during the incubation period of AIDS. Nature **362** 359–362

Falk K, Rotzschke O and Rammensee H-G (1990) Cellular peptide composition governed by major histocompatibility complex class I molecules. *Nature* **348** 248–251

Falk K, Rotzschke O, Stevanovic S, Jung G and Rammensee H-G (1991) Allele specific motifs revealed by sequencing of self peptides eluted from MHC molecules. *Nature* **351** 290–296

Fremont DH, Matsumura M, Stura EA, Peterson PA and Wilson IA (1992) Crystal structures of two viral peptides in complex with murine MHC class I H-2Kb. *Science* **257** 919–927

Goldberg AL and Rock KL (1992) Proteolysis, proteosomes and antigen presentation. *Nature* **357** 375–379

Gotch FM, Kelly C, Ellis SA *et al* (1985) Characterisation of the HLA A2.2 subtype: further evidence for heterogeneity. *Immunogenetics* **21** 11–23

Gotch FM, Nixon DF, Alp N, McMichael AJ and Borysiewicz LK (1990) High frequency of memory and effector gag specific cytotoxic T lymphocytes in HIV seropositive individuals. *International Immunology* **2** 707–712

Guo H-C, Jardetzky TS, Garrett TP, Lane WS, Strominger JL and Wiley DC (1992) Different

length peptides bind to HLA Aw68 similarly at their ends but bulge out in the middle. *Nature* **360** 364–360
Hill AV, Elvin J, Willis AC *et al* (1992) Molecular analysis of the association of HLA-B53 and resistance to severe malaria. *Nature* **360** 434–439
Hoffenbach A, Langlade-Demoyen P, Dadaglio G *et al* (1989) Unusually high frequencies of HIV-specific cytotoxic T lymphocytes in humans. *Journal of Immunology* **142** 452–462
Holmes EC, Zhang LQ, Simmonds P, Ludlam CA and Leigh-Brown AJ Convergent and divergent sequence evolution in the surface envelope glycoprotein of human immunodeficiency virus type I within a single infected patient. *Proceedings of the National Academy of Science* **89** 4835–4839
Hunt DF, Henderson RA, Shabanowitz J *et al* (1992) Characterization of peptides bound to the class I MHC molecule HLA A2.1 by mass spectometry. *Science* **255** 1261–1263
Jacobson S, Shida H, McFarlin DE, Fauci AS and Koenig S (1990) Circulating CD8+ cytotoxic T lymphocytes to HTLV-I pX in patients with HTLV-I associated neurological disease. *Nature* **348** 245–248
Jameson SC, Carbone FR and Bevan MJ (1993) Clone-specific T cell receptor antagonists of major histocompatibility complex class I-restricted cytotoxic T cells. *Journal of Experimental Medicine* **177** 1541–15050
Kaslow R, Duquensoy R, Van Raden M *et al* (1990) A1,Cw7,B8,DR3 HLA antigen combination associated with rapid decline of T-helper lymphocytes in HIV-1 infection. *Lancet* **335** 927–30
Klenerman P, Rowland-Jones S, McAdam S *et al* (1994) Naturally occurring HIV-1 gag variants antagonise cytotoxic T cell activity. *Nature* **369** 403–407
McCune JM (1991) HIV-1: the infective process in vivo. *Cell* **64** 351–363
McMichael A, Gotch F and Rothbard J (1986) HLA B37 determines an influenza A virus nucleoprotein epitope recognized by cytotoxic T lymphocytes. *Journal of Experimental Medicine* **164** 1397–1406
Macatonia SE, Lau R, Patterson S, Pinching AJ and Knight SC (1990) Dendritic cell infection, depletion and dysfunction in HIV infected individuals. *Immunology* **71** 38–45
Mallal S, Cameron PU, French MAH and Dawkins RL (1990) MHC genes and HIV infection. *Lancet* **335** 1591–1592
Mann DL, Marray C, Yarchoan R, Blattner WA and Goedert JJ (1988) HLA antigen frequencies in HIV-1 seropositive disease-free individuals and patients with AIDS. *Journal of AIDS* **1** 13–17
Michalek MT, Grant EP, Gramm C, Goldberg AL and Rock KL (1993) A role for the ubiquitin-dependent proteolytic pathway in MHC class I-restricted antigen presentation. *Nature* **363** 552–554
Moskaphidis D, Lechner F, Pircher H and Zinkernagel RM (1993) Virus persistence in acutely infected immunocompetent mice by exhaustion of antiviral cytotoxic effector T cells. *Nature* **362** 758
Myers G, Korber B, Berzofsky JA, Smith RF and Pavlakis GN (eds) (1992) *Human Retroviruses and AIDS 1992* Los Alamos National Laboratory, Los Alamos, New Mexico
Neefjes J, Momberg F and Hammerling G (1993) Selective and ATP-dependent translocation of peptides by the MHC-encoded transporter. *Science* **261** 769–771
Nixon DF, Townsend ARM, Elvin JG, Rizza CR, Gallwey J and McMichael AJ (1988) HIV-1 gag-specific cytotoxic T lymphocytes defined with recombinant vaccinia virus and synthetic peptides. *Nature* **336** 484–487
Nowak MA, Anderson RM, McLean AR, Wolfs TFW, Goudsmit J and May RM (1991) Antigenic diversity thresholds and the development of AIDS. *Science* **254** 963–969
Pantaleo G, Graziosi C, Demarest JF *et al* (1993) HIV infection is active and progressive in lymphoid tissue during the clinically latent stage of disease. *Nature* **362** 355–358
Peterlin BM and Luciw PA (1988) Molecular biology of HIV. *AIDS* **2 (Supplement 1)** S29–S40

Phillips RE, Rowland-Jones S, Nixon DF *et al* (1991) Human immunodeficiency virus genetic variation that can escape cytotoxic T cell recognition. *Nature* **354** 453–459

Plata F, Autran B, Martins L P *et al* (1987) AIDS virus specific cytotoxic T lymphocytes in lung disorders. *Nature* **328** 348–351

Rotzschke O and Falk K (1991) Naturally-occurring peptide antigens derived from the MHC class-I-restricted processing pathway. *Immunology Today* **12** 447–455

Shepherd JC, Schumacher TNM, Ashton-Rickardt PG *et al* (1993) TAP 1-dependent peptide translocation in vitro is ATP dependent and peptide selective. *Cell* **74** 577–584

Steel CM, Ludlum C, Beatson D *et al* (1988) HLA haplotype A1 B8 DR3 as a risk factor for HIV-related disease. *Lancet* **i** 1185–1188

Townsend A and Trowsdale J (1993) The transporters associated with antigen presentation. *Seminars in Cell Biology* **4** 53–61

Townsend ARM, McMichael AJ and Brownlee GG (1985) *Recognition of the Viral Nucleoprotein by Influenza A Specific Cytotoxic T Cells,* Humana Press, London

Townsend A, Rothbard J, Gotch F, Bahadur B, Wraith D and McMichael A (1986) The epitopes of influenza nucleoprotein recognized by cytotoxic T lymphocytes can be defined with short synthetic peptides. *Cell* **44** 959–968

Townsend A, Elliott T, Cerundolo V, Foster L, Barber B and Tse A (1990) Assembly of MHC class I molecules analyzed in vitro. *Cell* **62** 285–295

Van Bleek GM and Nathenson SM (1990) Isolation of an endogenously processed immunodominant viral peptide from the class I H2Kb molecule. *Nature* **348** 213

Wain-Hobson S (1993) Viral burden and AIDS. *Nature* **366** 22

Walker DB, Chakrabati S, Moss B *et al* (1987) HIV specific cytotoxic T lymphocytes in seropositive individuals. *Nature* **328** 345–348

Zhang W, Young AC, Imarai M, Nathenson SG and Sacchettini JC (1992) Crystal structure of the major histocompatibility complex class I H-2Kb molecule containing a single viral peptide: implications for peptide binding and T-cell receptor recognition. *Proceedings of the National Academy of Sciences of the USA* **89** 8403–8407

Zinkernagel RM and Doherty PC (1974) Immunological surveillance against altered self components by sensitised T lympocytes in lymphocytic choriomeningitis. *Nature* **251** 547

Zinkernagel RM and Doherty PC (1979) MHC-restricted cytotoxic T cells: studies on the biological role of polymorphic major transplantation antigens determining T cell restriction-specificty, function and responsiveness. *Advances in Immunology* **27** 51–177

The authors are responsible for the accuracy of the references.

# Accessory Signals for Growth and Differentiation of Human T Lymphocytes

**STEFAN C MEUER • YVONNE SAMSTAG • BURKHART SCHRAVEN**
*Applied Immunology, Deutsches Krebsforschungszentrum, D-69120 Heidelberg, Germany*



## INTRODUCTION

Resting T lymphocytes having received an initial triggering signal through the antigen receptor/CD3 (T cell receptor [TCR]/CD3) complex require additional signals to differentiate into immunoregulatory and effector lymphocytes (Schwartz, 1990; Jenkins, 1992). Such accessory signals—also called co-stimulatory signals—are transmitted through a large number of accessory receptor types expressed in the lymphocyte plasma membrane. Due to the availability of monoclonal antibodies and molecular cloning techniques, there is now sufficient information on the structural characteristics of these glycoproteins. In addition, in a considerable number of cases, endogenous ligand molecules have also been identified and characterized. Accessory receptors belong to large superfamilies of molecules including the Ig superfamily, integrins, and selectins (Emmrich *et al*, 1986; Samstag *et al*, 1988; Geppert *et al*, 1990; June *et al*, 1990). Altogether they form a complex system that in addition to its tremendous structural heterogeneity, is further complicated by dynamic regulatory mechanisms. The latter influence cell surface density, conformation, structural features through alternative splicing mechanisms and the generation of soluble receptor variants. Such alterations are induced by external stimuli (eg cytokines) and are transient.

## T CELL RECEPTOR CONTROL OF ACCESSORY RECEPTOR SIGNALLING

Given that cellular immune reactions are antigen specific, signals transmitted through accessory receptors must be controlled by the T cell receptor for antigen. How is this control exerted?

To investigate this question, resting human T lymphocytes were exposed to monoclonal antibodies directed at both the T cell receptor complex and a

*Cancer Surveys* Volume 22: *Molecular Mechanisms of the Immune Response*

series of accessory receptors all expressed on the T cell surface. As shown in Fig. 1, none of these monoclonal antibodies alone is capable of inducing T cell proliferation (an exception is certain monoclonal antibodies directed at CD2). Following overnight incubation, each sample was then challenged with a combination of monoclonal antibodies directed at the CD2 glycoprotein, an accessory receptor that is expressed only by T lymphocytes and natural killer cells. The result of this experiment, which is shown in Fig. 1, suggests a number of facts about its function.

(a) Binding of the antigen receptor CD3 complex by a single ligand (here a monoclonal antibody exerting an antigen like effect) is itself not sufficient to induce T cell growth.
(b) Antibodies directed at accessory receptors—in the absence of T cell receptor stimulation—do not produce detectable activation signals.
(c) Exceptions to step b are certain antibodies directed at CD2 that have a unique capacity to induce the expression of the functional T cell repertoire including DNA synthesis (Meuer *et al,* 1983; Bierer *et al,* 1988) (until now, no receptor structure other than CD2 has been identified through which, in the absence of antigen receptor triggering, T cell activation is mediated). The fact that T cells can be triggered through CD2 (Meuer *et al,* 1984) provided the first evidence for the notion that accessory structures may function as receptors.
(d) Binding of the T cell receptor by a single ligand, albeit incapable of inducing lymphocyte activation itself, is, however, not a neutral event (Meuer *et al,* 1984; Meuer and Meyer zum Büschenfelde, 1986; Lamb *et al,* 1987). Thus, when T lymphocytes are pretreated with an antigen like monoclonal antibody for several hours prior to their exposure to mitogenic CD2 antibodies no longer respond to CD2 triggering but become unresponsive. Importantly, the cell surface expression of CD2 remains unaltered. Therefore, one has to conclude that intracellular events related to the signalling function of CD2 must change through binding of the antigen receptor alone.

The experimental system described here provides a means to study interactions between the T cell receptor and CD2 receptor complexes by comparing molecular compositions in the CD2 responsive versus the CD2 unresponsive state. Since in general the typical cell surface receptors of the immune system require molecular interactions with additional molecules to fulfil their signalling functions (Veillette *et al,* 1988; Schraven *et al,* 1990, 1991; Chalupny *et al,* 1991; Glaichenhaus *et al,* 1991; Beyers *et al,* 1992), the question was asked which molecules associate with CD2 and can alterations be observed in the CD2 associated signalling molecules in the anergic, CD2 unresponsive state?

CD2 immunoprecipitates were obtained and subjected to in vitro kinase reactions during which—if protein kinases are associated with the precipitated

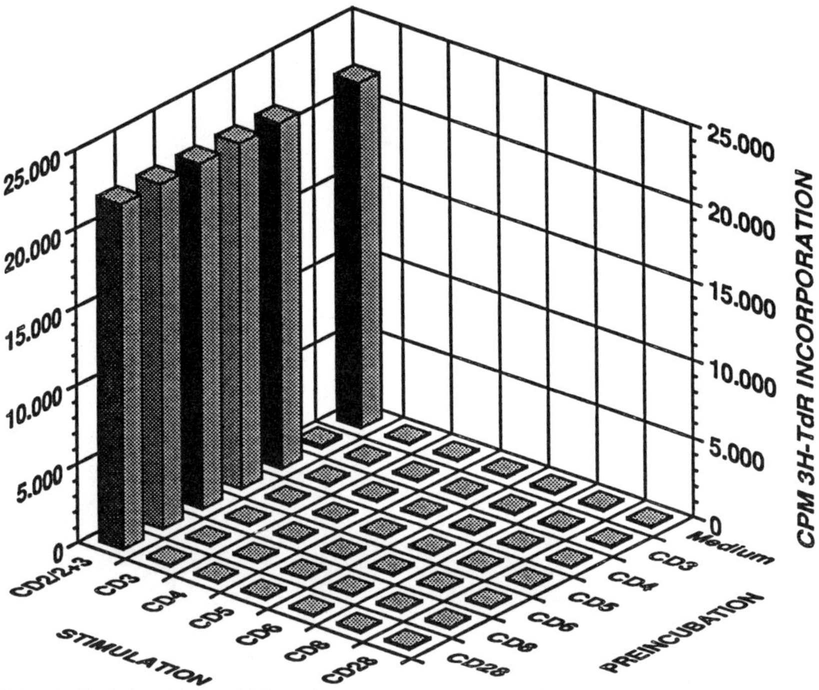


**Fig. 1.** Peripheral blood T lymphocytes were exposed to monoclonal antibodies directed at cell surface receptors and medium as indicated (stimulation). Concomitantly, another set of T cells was preincubated with monoclonal antibodies directed at receptors as indicated (preincubation) overnight and subsequently challenged with a mitogenic concentration of monoclonal antibodies directed at the CD2 receptor. As shown, although preincubation with antibodies directed at accessory receptors does not influence subsequent responsiveness to CD2 triggering preincubation with CD3 monoclonal antibodies induces an unresponsive state

molecule—substrate molecules undergo $^{32}$P phosphorylation. These can then be detected following two dimensional gel electrophoresis by subsequent autoradiography. Here, their identity was analysed by means of re-precipitation experiments using specific antisera directed at known signalling proteins. As shown in Fig. 2, apart from two as yet unknown and undefined molecules of 32 kDa and 29 kDa (reducing conditions), respectively, a number of known molecules associate with CD2. These include the tyrosine phosphatase CD45, two tyrosine kinases of the *src* family, namely p56$^{lck}$ and p59$^{fyn}$, and most importantly, two subunits of the T cell antigen receptor complex, namely the ζ and ε molecules. These two molecules have been clearly demonstrated to have a central role in cell signalling through transmembrane receptors in lymphocytes and to contain sequence motifs responsible for this function (Brown *et al,* 1989; Monostori *et al,* 1990; Spruyt *et al,* 1991; Howard *et al,* 1992; Moingeon *et al,* 1992; Wegener *et al,* 1992). They would represent ideal candidates for functional components through which antigen receptor and the accessory receptor CD2 could be linked. With regard to ζ, it is known that this

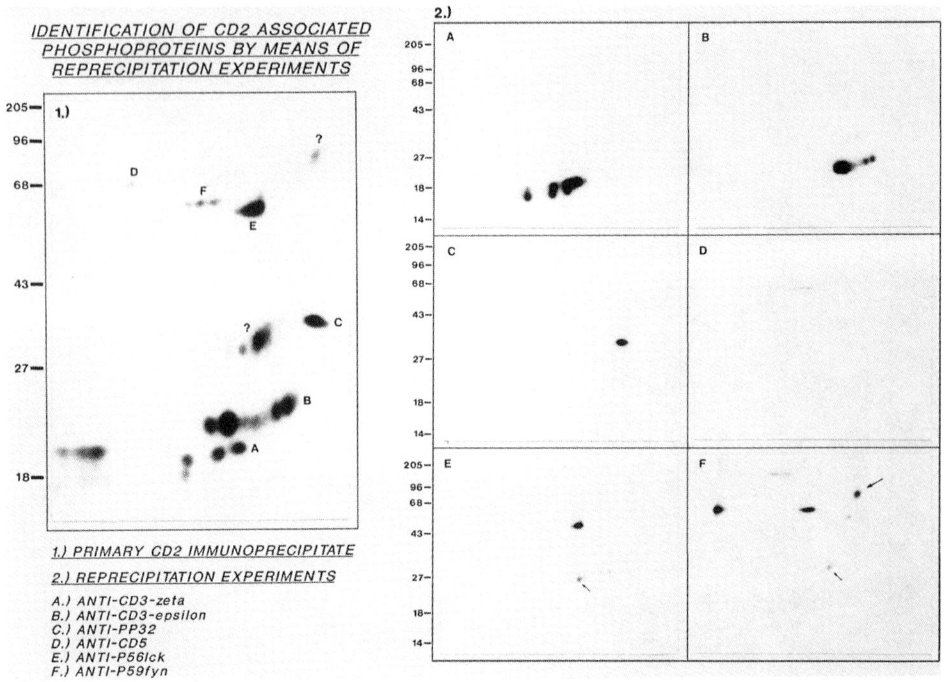


**Fig. 2.** Identification of CD2 associated proteins by means of in vitro kinase assay reaction of a CD2 immunoprecipitate. Note that CD2 and CD45 are themselves not visible under these conditions. The co-precipitated proteins were identified by means of re-precipitation experiments using specific antisera. The figure shows an autoradiograph

signalling component not only does associate with the T cell receptor, but also appears in association with the Fc receptor γIII (CD16) in CD3/TCR negative natural killer (Anderson *et al,* 1992) cells, suggesting redundancy regarding its potential association with lymphocyte receptors.

Does the CD2 complex possess its own associated ζ and ε molecules or does it share them with the T cell antigen receptor? To investigate this, we took advantage of the fact that it is possible to remove the T cell receptor and its associated molecules from the cell surface by modulation. If T cell receptor and CD2 shared the identical ζ and ε chains, then, following T cell receptor modulation and loss from the cell surface, ζ and ε chains should no longer be associated with CD2. On the other hand, if CD2 had its own signalling molecules, then T cell receptor modulation should not affect the CD2 associated ζ and ε chains. Figure 3 shows that the first possibility is correct. Thus, following removal of the antigen receptor from the T cell surface, the specific associations of CD2 with ζ and ε are lost. Note, however, that TCR/CD3 modulated cells still contain a large pool of ζ chains (not shown). This demonstrates that only a proportion of the cellular ζ (and ε) pool associates with the T cell antigen receptor and that these same molecules are apparently also linked to the CD2 complex. Interestingly, the as yet unknown 29 kDa phosphoprotein is also no longer detectable in TCR/CD3 modulated cells (Schraven *et al,* 1993).

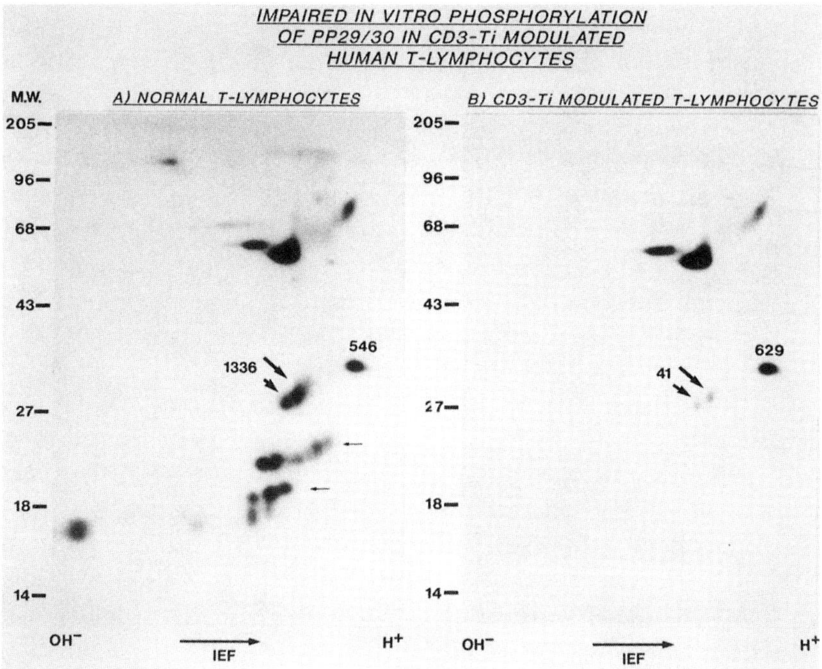


**Fig. 3.** Comparison of the composition of the CD2 molecular complex in untreated v. T cell receptor CD3 modulated human T cells. Note that the ζ and ε chains of the T cell receptor are uncoupled from CD2 in the CD2 unresponsive state. Moreover, a 29/30 kDa dimer (under reducing conditions) disappears in response to this treatment. (Numbers represent integrated density units.) Additional co-precipitating proteins such as $p56^{lck}$, $p59^{fyn}$ and pp32 are not altered in the course of T cell receptor modulation

Whether this results from impaired phosphorylation (loss of a TCR associated kinase) or structural co-modulation is not known. Note that p29 (a disulphide linked dimer of 58 kDa) is expressed in natural killer cells—like ζ (Anderson *et al,* 1992)—as well (not shown).

Once the CD2 association with ζ and ε is lost, then this receptor complex can no longer fulfil a signalling function for growth induction. Uncoupling ζ and ε from CD2 therefore characterizes the CD2 unresponsive state, at least with regard to interleukin 2 (IL2) production and proliferation. This does not necessarily exclude other responses being induced through CD2. However, these are unrelated to the mechanisms underlying clonal T cell expansion as detected by measuring DNA synthesis.

## THE QUALITY OF AN ACCESSORY SIGNAL IN LYMPHOCYTE ACTIVATION

Are there qualitative differences between T cell receptor mediated (primary) signals and accessory receptor mediated co-stimulatory (secondary) signals? The first evidence for differential qualities of T cell receptor versus accessory receptor mediated signalling events in T cells came from studies in which the functional responses of lymphocytes, triggered either through the antigen receptor alone or through co-aggregated accessory receptor molecules such as CD4 and CD8 or through the accessory receptor CD2, were compared (Emmrich *et al,* 1986; Samstag *et al,* 1988). It was found that whereas antigen receptor triggering alone was sufficient to produce IL2 receptor expression and production of γ interferon, the induction of IL2 synthesis and secretion was clearly dependent on an accessory receptor mediated signalling event. The same holds true for the induction of responsiveness to monokines such as IL1 and IL6, which can only be observed in T cells that have received an accessory receptor dependent signal (Endler-Jobst *et al,* 1991).

Given these observations, it seemed justified to search for intracellular signalling events that were specifically related to accessory receptors. To this end, resting human T lymphocytes were obtained, prelabelled with $^{32}P$ orthophosphate and subsequently triggered through either CD3 or CD2 using an appropriate set of monoclonal antibodies. Subsequently, postnuclear lysates were obtained, and molecules were separated in two dimensional gel electrophoresis and then compared by means of autoradiography. The two dimensional gels shown in Fig. 4 demonstrate two major differences that represent specific signalling events related to triggering of the accessory receptor CD2. Thus, there is de novo phosphorylation of a 67 kDa cytoplasmic protein. With similar kinetics, dephosphorylation of a 19 kDa protein occurs in T cells. Phosphorylation of p67 and dephosphorylation of pp19 (Samstag *et al,* 1992) correlate with late functional events (previously known to be inducible only through accessory receptor triggering), namely IL2 synthesis and IL6 responsiveness, but not with the induction of the γ interferon gene. CD2 is not the only accessory receptor through which these changes can be induced. Thus, co-cross linking of CD4 or CD8 to the T cell receptor results in analogous responses (Fig. 5). The mode of T cell triggering through CD2 by monoclonal antibodies therefore could be interpreted as providing primary plus secondary signals simultaneously.

Isoelectric focusing of p67 showed that its molecular weight and mobility resembled that of the cytoplasmic protein L-plastin/fimbrin (de Arruda *et al,* 1990; Zu *et al,* 1990), which was confirmed using specific antisera. Fimbrin represents an actin binding protein, which in addition expresses calmodulin binding motifs and calcium binding sites, suggesting functions that influence the conformation of cytoskeletal components as well as signalling properties. It is not unlikely that these activities are regulated through phosphorylation and therefore can be modulated through accessory receptors.

The identity of pp19 was determined following its purification from preparative two dimensional gels and microsequencing. Four internal peptide sequences were identified and demonstrated that pp19 expressed by human T cells exhibits complete sequence homology with the recently cloned small actin binding protein, cofilin (Ohta *et al,* 1989; Ogawa *et al,* 1990). Peptide sequences were used to prepare antisera specifically to recognize cofilin. By

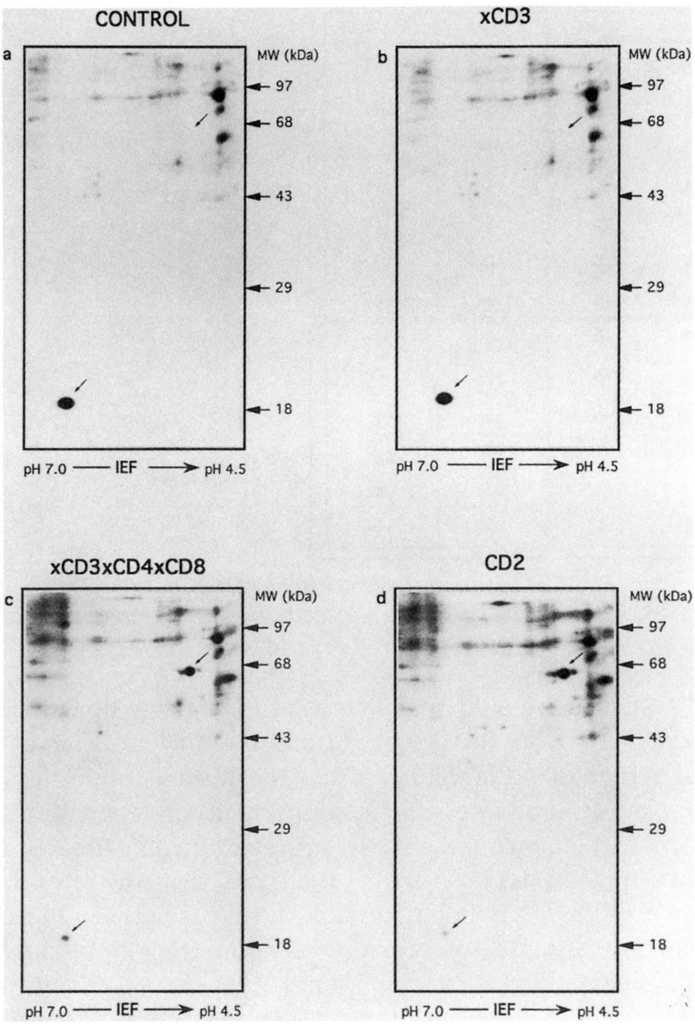


**Fig. 4.** Triggering resting human T cells through accessory receptors induces phosphorylation of a 67 kDa protein (arrows in the upper right corners) and concomitant dephosphorylation of a 19 kDa phosphoprotein (lower left corners). By contrast, triggering the T cell receptor by cross linked CD3 antibodies alone does not alter the phosphorylation state of pp19 and p67. Importantly, secretion of γ interferon occurs to a virtually identical extent in all stimulated cultures including CD3 stimulated cells, thus demonstrating that the antibodies exhibit analogous intrinsic triggering activity

employing these reagents and cell fractionation techniques, it became clear that cofilin dephosphorylation was associated with its subsequent translocation into the nuclear compartment, suggesting that cofilin might represent a mediator of accessory signals from the cytoplasm into the nucleus. The functional significance of the cofilin translocation, which appears to be mediated through a nuclear translocation signal sequence (KKRKK), is not known at present. However, from earlier studies which demonstrated that cofilin alters the conformation of actin from polymeric F-actin to oligomeric or monomeric

| | CD3xCD3 | CD3xCD4 | CD3xCD8 | CD3+MO | CD2+CD2 | |
|---|---|---|---|---|---|---|
| $Ca^{2+}$↑ | + | + | + | + | + | $1^0$ Signal |
| IP3 ↑ | + | + | + | + | + | |
| PKC activ. | + | + | + | + | + | |
| ζ-Phos. | + | + | + | + | + | |
| pp29/32 shift | + | + | + | + | + | |
| IL2-Resp. | + | + | + | + | + | |
| IFN-γSecr. | + | + | + | + | + | |
| IL1-Resp. | − | + | + | + | + | + $2^0$ Signal |
| IL6-Resp. | − | + | + | + | + | |
| IL2-Secr. | − | + | + | + | + | |
| $p56^{lck}$ shift | − | + | + | + | + | |
| cofilin dephos. | − | + | + | + | + | |
| l-plastin phosph. | − | + | + | + | + | |

**Fig. 5.** Early and late lymphocyte responses following stimulation through various cell surface receptors. A variety of responses are strictly dependent on an accessory signal for T cell activation

G-actin (Nishida *et al,* 1984), one could speculate that cofilin functions as a transporter of monomeric actin from the cytoplasm into the nuclear compartment. The presence of actin/cofilin complexes inside the nucleus indicates a functional quality of this event: monomeric actin supports accurate transcription of RNA polymerase II (Scheer *et al,* 1984) and at the same time is a potent inhibitor of DNase I (Peitsch *et al,* 1993), an enzyme that was recently demonstrated to be involved in DNA fragmentation during apoptosis. Thus, cofilin/actin translocation in response to accessory receptor triggering could promote transcriptional events and block apoptosis—that is, represent a growth and survival mechanism of T cells. There is yet no formal proof to support this hypothesis. Nevertheless, there is further evidence to support such a view:

(a) In malignant T cells (cells that do not die), there is a constitutive translocation of actin/cofilin complexes from the cytosol into the nucleus, indicating that the accessory receptor dependent signalling pathway described is out of control. This may be related to the prolonged lifespan of malignant cells.
(b) Activation of untransformed T cells through CD2 reduces their sensitivity towards antibody induced apoptosis under certain experimental conditions (Klas *et al,* 1993).
(c) Inhibition of cofilin dephosphorylation by ocadaic acid inhibits the transcription of the *IL2* gene but not of the γ interferon gene (not shown).

The molecular basis of these phenomena and their relationship to the pp19 molecule are now amenable to analysis.

## SUMMARY

Accessory signals represent the level at which functional immune responses are regulated. Impairment of ligand-receptor interactions or, alternatively, intracellular signalling processes plays a pivotal part in vivo. Thus, tumour tolerance might result from missing co-stimulatory signals, which is supported by numerous recent data. Conversely, blocking accessory receptors might provide the means to influence allograft rejection. Upregulation of accessory receptors and their ligands is a hallmark of inflammatory reactions. Finally, given that particular microenvironments are characterized by the presence of particular combinations of ligand molecules for critical accessory receptors on T lymphocytes, one could envisage novel approaches to local immune intervention. All these perspectives, however, are based on our understanding of how accessory receptors are composed and interact with intracellular enzymes, which all together transmit critical signals to the nucleus, and on an understanding of how these signals contribute to functional T cell behaviour.


## References


Anderson PM, Caligiuri M, Ritz J and Schlossman SF (1992) CD3-negative natural killer cells express zeta TCR as a part of a novel molecular complex. *Nature* **341** 159–162

Beyers AD, Spruyt LL and Williams AF (1992) Molecular associations between the T-lymphocyte antigen receptor complex and the surface antigens CD2, CD4, or CD8 and CD5. *Proceedings of the National Academy of Sciences of the USA* **89** 2945–2949

Bierer BE, Peterson A, Gorga JC, Herrmann SH and Burakoff SJ (1988) Synergistic T cell activation via the physiological ligands for CD2 and the T cell receptor. *Journal of Experimental Medicine* **168** 1145–1156

Brown MH, Cantrell DA, Brattsand DJ, Crumpton MJ and Gullberg M (1989) The CD2 antigen associates with the T-cell antigen receptor CD3 complex on the surface of human T lymphocytes. *Nature* **339** 551–553

Chalupny NJ, Ledbetter JA and Kavathas P (1991) Association of CD8 with $p56^{lck}$ is required for early T cell signalling events. *EMBO Journal* **10** 1201–1207

de Arruda M, Watson S, Lin CS, Leavitt J and Matsudair P (1990) Fimbrin is a homologue of the cytoplasmic phosphoprotein plastin and has domains homologous with calmodulin and actin gelation proteins. *Journal of Cell Biology* **111** 1069–1079

Emmrich F, Strittmatter U and Eichmann K (1986) Synergism in the activation of human CD8 T cells by crosslinking the T cell receptor complex with the CD8 differentiation antigen. *Proceedings of the National Academy of Sciences of the USA* **83** 8298–8302

Endler-Jobst B, Schraven B, Hutmacher B and Meuer SC (1991) Human T cell responses to IL-1 and IL-6 are dependent on signals mediated through CD2. *J Immunol* **146** 1736–1742

Geppert TD, Davis LS, Gur H, Wacholtz MC and Lipsky PE (1990) Accessory cell signals involved in T-cell activation. *Immunological Reviews* **117** 5–66

Glaichenhaus N, Shastri N, Littman DR and Turner JM (1991) Requirement for association of $p56^{lck}$ with CD4 in antigen-specific signal transduction in T cells. *Cell* **64** 511–520

Howard FD, Moingeon P, Moebius U *et al* (1992) The CD3 zeta cytoplasmic domain mediates CD2-induced T-cell activation. *Journal of Experimental Medicine* **176** 139–145

Jenkins MK (1992) The role of cell division in the induction of clonal anergy. *Immunology Today* **13** 69–73

June CH, Ledbetter JA, Linsle PS and Thompson CB (1990) Role of the CD28 receptor in T-cell activation. *Immunology Today* **11** 211–216

Klas C, Debatin KM, Jonker RR and Krammer PH (1993) Activation interferes with the APO-1 pathway im mature human T cells. *International Immunology* **5** 625–630

Lamb JR, Zanders ED, Sewell W, Crumpton MJ, Feldmann M and Owen MJ (1987) Antigen-specific T-cell unresponsiveness in cloned helper T-cells mediated via the CD2 or CD3/Ti receptor pathways. *European Journal of Immunology* **17** 1641–1644

Meuer SC and Meyer zum Büschenfelde KH (1986) T cell receptor triggering induces responsiveness to interleukin 1 and interleukin 2 but does not lead to T cell proliferation. *Journal of Immunology* **136** 4106–4112

Meuer SC, Hodgdon JC, Hussey RE, Protentis JP, Schlossman SF and Reinherz EL (1983) Antigen-like effects of monoclonal antibodies directed at receptors on human T cell clones. *Journal of Experimental Medicine* **158** 988–993

Meuer SC, Hussey RE, Fabbi M *et al* (1984) Alternative pathway of T cell activation: a functional role for the 50kD T11 sheep erythrocyte receptor protein. *Cell* **36** 897–906

Moingeon P, Lucich JC, McConkey DJ *et al* (1992) CD3 zeta dependence of the CD2 pathway of activation in T lymphocytes and NK cells. *Proceedings of the National Academy of Sciences of the USA* **89** 1492–1496

Monostori E, Desai D, Brown MH, Cantrell DA and Crumpton MJ (1990) Activation of human T lymphocytes via the CD2 antigen results in tyrosine phosphorylation of T cell antigen receptor z-chains. *Journal of Immunology* **144** 1010–1016

Mueller DL, Jenkins MK and Schwartz R (1989) Clonal expansion versus functional clonal inactivation: a costimulatory signaling pathway determines the outcome of T cell antigen receptor occupancy. *Annual Review of Immunology* **7** 445–480

Nishida E, Maekawa S and Sakai H (1984) Cofilin, a protein in porcine brain that binds to actin filaments and inhibits their interactions with myosin and tropomyosin. *Biochemistry* **23** 5307–5313

Ogawa K, Tashima M, Yumoto Y *et al* (1990) Coding sequence of human placenta cofilin cDNA. *Nucleic Acids Research* **18** 7169

Ohta Y, Nishida E, Sakai H and Miyamoto E (1989) Dephosphorylation of cofilin accompanies heat shock induced nuclear accumulation of cofilin. *Proceedings of the National Academy of Sciences of the USA* **264** 16143–16148

Peitsch MC, Polzar B, Stephan H *et al* (1993) Characterization of the endogenous deoxyribonuclease involved in nuclear DNA degradation during apoptosis (programmed cell death). *EMBO Journal* **12** 371–377

Samstag Y, Emmrich F and Staehelin T (1988) Activation of human T lymphocytes: differential effects of CD3- and CD8-mediated signals. *Proceedings of the National Academy of Sciences of the USA* **85** 9689–9693

Samstag Y, Henning SW, Bader A and Meuer SC (1992) Dephosphorylation of pp19: a common second signal for human T cell activation mediated through different accessory molecules. *International Immunology* **4** 1255–1261

Scheer U, Hinssen H, Franke WW and Jockusch BM (1984) Microinjection of actin-binding proteins and actin antibodies demonstrates involvement of nuclear actin in transcription of lampbrush chromosomes. *Cell* **39** 111–122

Schraven B, Samstag Y, Altevog P and Meuer SC (1990) Association of CD2 and CD45 on human T lymphocytes. *Nature* **345** 71–74

Schraven B, Kirchgessner H, Gaber B, Samstag Y and Meuer SC (1991) A functional complex is formed in human T lymphocytes between the protein tyrosine phosphatase CD45, the protein tyrosine kinase $p56^{lck}$, and pp32, a possible common substrate. *European Journal of Immunology* **21** 2469–2477

Schraven B, Wild M, Kirchgessner H *et al* (1993) Alterations of CD2 association with T cell receptor signaling molecules in "CD2 unresponsive" human T lymphocytes. *European Journal of Immunology* **23** 119–123

Schwartz RH (1990) A cell culture model for T lymphocyte clonal anergy. *Science* **248** 1349

Spruyt LL, Glennie MJ, Beyers AD and Williams AF (1991) Signal transduction by the CD2 antigen in T cells and natural killer cells requirement for expression of a functional T cell receptor or binding of antibody Fc to the Fc receptor, Fc gamma RIIIA (CD16). *Journal of Experimental Medicine* **174** 1407–1416

Veillette A, Bookman MA, Horak EM and Bolen JB (1988) The CD4 and CD8 T cell surface antigens are associated with the internal membrane tyrosine-protein kinase $p56^{lck}$. *Cell* **55** 301–308

Wegener AM, Letourneur KF, Hoelver A, Brocker T, Luton F and Malissen B (1992) The T cell receptor/CD3 complex is composed of at least two autonomous transduction molecules. *Cell* **68** 83–95

Zu Y, Shigesada K, Nishida E *et al* (1990) 65-kilodalton protein phosphorylated by interleukin 2 stimulation bears two putative actin-binding sites and two calcium-binding sites. *Biochemistry* **29** 8319–8324

The authors are responsible for the accuracy of the references.

# Regulation and Function of p21 ras in T Lymphocytes

M IZQUIERDO PASTOR • M WOODROW • D CANTRELL

*Lymphocyte Activation Laboratory, Imperial Cancer Research Fund, 44 Lincoln's Inn Fields, London WC2A 3PX*



## INTRODUCTION

The term "T cell activation" refers to the events triggered by antigen stimulation that culminate in the production of cytokines such as interleukin 2 (IL2) and the expression of cytokine receptors such as the IL2 receptor (Crabtree, 1989; Janeway and Golstein, 1992). The physiological trigger for T cell activation is engagement of the T cell antigen receptor (TCR) with antigen/major histocompatibility molecules presented to the T cell on the surface of an antigen presenting cell. The TCR is a multichain complex consisting of a disulphide linked heterodimer of the idiotypic α and β chains noncovalently associated with a signal transduction complex composed of the invariant CD3 γ, δ and ε chains and the ζ and η subunits (Reth, 1989; Weissman *et al,* 1989; Weiss, 1993). Triggering of the TCR/CD3 complex initiates a cascade of biochemical events, the earliest of which is activation of intracellular protein tyrosine kinases (PTKs) (Klausner and Samelson, 1991). This activation of PTKs appears to be absolutely required for all subsequent T cell responses (June *et al,* 1990). Protein tyrosine kinases are known to couple the TCR to an inositol lipid specific phospholipase C, PLCγ1 (Weiss *et al,* 1991), thus enabling the TCR to regulate the hydrolysis of membrane phosphoinositides, releasing inositol polyphosphates, which regulate intracellular $Ca^{2+}$, and diacylglycerols, which activate the serine/threonine kinase, protein kinase C (PKC) (Nishizuka, 1988; Berridge and Irvine, 1989; Berry and Nishizuka, 1989).

A second PTK controlled signalling pathway to originate from the TCR involves the guanine nucleotide binding proteins $p21^{ras}$ (Downward *et al,* 1990, 1992a). The RAS proteins bind GTP and have an intrinsic GTPase activity that

*Cancer Surveys* Volume 22: *Molecular Mechanisms of the Immune Response*

catalyzes the hydrolysis of GTP to GDP. A consensus from RAS studies is that the GTP bound form of the protein is the biologically active form (Satoh *et al,* 1992). In T cells stimulated via the TCR, the RAS proteins rapidly accumulate in the active GTP bound state. Activation of PKC with phorbol esters or diacylglycerols also induces the accumulation of RAS-GTP complexes. Regulation of $p21^{ras}$ by PKC appears to be cell lineage specific, since it occurs in T cells but not in other haemopoietic cells such as mast cells or myeloid cells (Downward *et al,* 1992a). However, the functional relevance of PKC for receptor coupling to RAS is not clear. In particular, PKC does not couple the TCR to $p21^{ras}$, and instead a PKC independent pathway involving PTKs has a critical role in TCR regulation of RAS (Izquierdo *et al,* 1992). The realization that $Ca^{2+}$ and PKC do not couple the TCR to RAS is important because it indicates that at least two signalling pathways can originate from the TCR, one mediated by PLCγ1 and the other by RAS (Fig. 1).

## REGULATION OF THE RAS-GUANINE NUCLEOTIDE BINDING CYCLE

The level of active $p21^{ras}$-GTP complexes is determined by a balance between the rate of hydrolysis of bound GTP and the rate of exchange of bound GDP for cytosolic GTP (Downward, 1992). The GTPase activity of $p21^{ras}$ is controlled by GTPase activating proteins (GAPs), of which two mammalian proteins are known, p120-GAP and neurofibromin (McCormick, 1989; Ballester *et al,* 1990). Proteins that regulate guanine nucleotide exchange on RAS have also been characterized, and in mammalian cells, they include the homologues of the yeast CDC25 protein and the *Drosophila* "son of sevenless" gene product, SOS (Bowtell *et al,* 1992; Shou *et al,* 1992). The proto-oncogene VAV has been described as an exchange protein for $p21^{ras}$ in T cells, although its structure suggests that it is more likely to be a rho/rac exchange protein (Adams *et al,* 1992; Gulbins *et al,* 1993).

The alternative mechanisms that could couple the TCR to RAS are TCR stimulation of $p21^{ras}$-guanine nucleotide exchange or TCR inhibition of RAS-GAP proteins. Experiments to explore RAS regulatory mechanisms have shown that TCR triggering inhibits the activity of RAS-GAP (Downward *et al,* 1990; Graves *et al,* 1991). It is not yet known which GAP protein, ie p120-GAP or neurofibromin, is the target for TCR regulation, nor is the mechanism that allows the TCR to inhibit RAS-GAP proteins understood, although PTKs are clearly involved in some way (Izquierdo *et al,* 1992). It has also been suggested that PTKs may allow the TCR to regulate a putative RAS exchange protein, VAV (Hunter and Karin, 1992). In fibroblasts, growth factors such as the epidermal growth factor (EGF) regulate $p21^{ras}$ by stimulating RAS-guanine nucleotide exchange (Buday and Downward, 1993b; Medema *et al,* 1993). The RAS exchange protein in fibroblasts is the mammalian homologue of the *Drosophila* SOS gene product (Egan *et al,* 1993; McCormick, 1993). The SOS protein is recruited to the activated EGF receptor cytoplasmic domain and

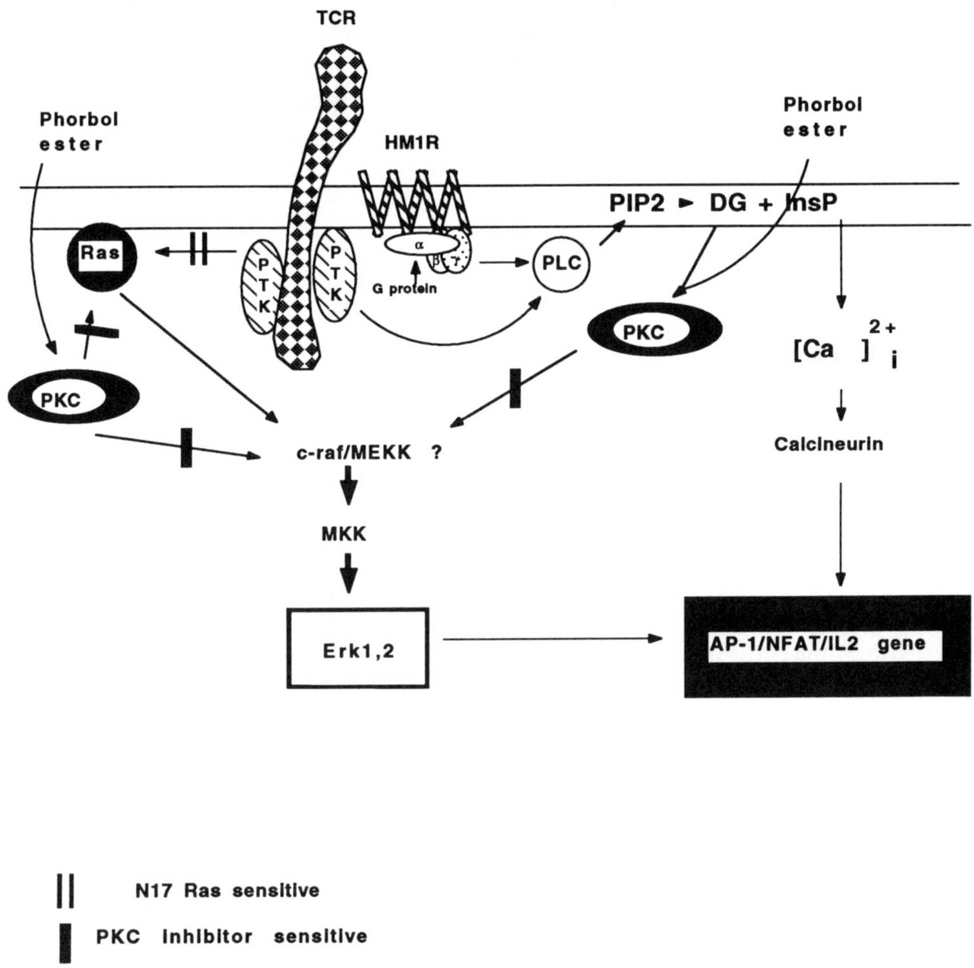


**Fig. 1.** Possible signalling pathways originating from the T cell antigen receptor. One such pathway is mediated by RAS proteins, another by PLCγ1. Erk1,2 = extracellular signal regulated kinases 1 and 2, HMIR = human muscarinic receptor type 1, $PIP_2$ = phosphatidyl inositol biphosphate, DG = diacylglycerol, InsP = inositol polyphosphates, MKK = MAP kinase kinase

hence to the cell membrane by the adapter protein GRB2/SEM5 (Buday and Downward, 1993a). T cells express GRB2 and SOS, but as yet nothing is known about their regulation and function (Buday L, Downward J, personal communication). Neither is it known whether the reported stimulatory effect of TCR induced tyrosine phosphorylation on the guanine nucleotide exchange activity of VAV has a major regulatory effect on $p21^{ras}$ in vivo.

## FUNCTION OF RAS, CALCIUM AND PKC IN T CELL ACTIVATION

Major breakthroughs in understanding signal transduction in T cells have been achieved because of co-ordinated efforts to link up immediate biochemical events triggered at the cell membrane with the transcription factors that control *IL2* gene expression. Interleukin 2 is encoded by a single gene, whose transcriptional activity is rapidly increased in activated T cells. Several studies have located a 267 bp transcriptional enhancer 5′ to the transcriptional initiation site of the *IL2* gene. Multiple ubiquitous transcription factors such as AP1, NFKB and OCT1 interact with this enhancer (Durand *et al,* 1987; Crabtree, 1989; Emmel *et al,* 1989). There are also binding sites for a unique lymphocyte specific transcriptional complex termed NFAT (nuclear factor of activated T cells), which appears to determine the T cell specificity and inducibility of *IL2* gene expression (Verweij *et al,* 1990). The signal transduction mechanisms that couple the TCR or accessory molecules to the transcription factors that interact with the *IL2* gene enhancer have become a paradigm of T cell activation.

Calcium and PKC are known to be important intracellular signals in T cell activation because pharmacological agents that elevate intracellular calcium (calcium ionophores) or stimulate PKC (phorbol esters) can mimic the TCR and induce T cell activation as judged by *IL2* gene expression (Weiss and Imboden, 1987; Cantrell *et al,* 1988). $p21^{ras}$ has a crucial function in T cells, as was shown by transient transfection protocols that examined the consequences of expressing mutated constitutively active or dominant inhibitory RAS mutants on T cell activation. The *RAS* oncogene $p21^{v\text{-}Ha\ ras}$ is mutated at codons 12 (Ser>Val) and 59 (Ala>Thr). These mutations render the RAS protein insensitive to negative regulation by RAS-GAP so that it accumulates in cells in an "active" GTP bound state. A second *RAS* mutant, $N17^{ras}$, blocks cytoplasmic RAS function by competing for RAS-guanine nucleotide exchange proteins, thereby preventing endogenous RAS activation by stopping exchange of GTP onto cytoplasmic RAS (Buday and Downward, 1993). $p21^{v\text{-}Ha\ ras}$, when expressed in T cells, can synergize with a calcium signal to activate the *IL2* gene (Baldari *et al,* 1992; Rayter *et al,* 1992). By contrast, expression of $N17^{ras}$ inhibits TCR induction of the *IL2* gene, indicating that RAS function is essential for TCR signal transduction (Rayter *et al,* 1992).

Multiple transcriptional factors regulate the *IL2* gene, but RAS regulation of the *IL2* gene is mediated in part by control of the transcriptional factor NFAT (Woodrow *et al,* 1993b). This factor has long been the focus of signal transduction studies in T cells because the immunosuppressive drugs cyclosporin A and FK506, which are widely used therapeutically in transplantation procedures, appear to regulate T cell activation via regulation of NFAT function (Emmel *et al,* 1989). Expression of the *IL2* gene cannot be induced by induction of a single signalling pathway but requires the action of several pathways that integrate at the level of the transcriptional factors that bind to the *IL2* enhancer. Studies of NFAT regulation have revealed how such integration of signals occurs: thus, NFAT is a heterodimer consisting of an AP1 component, found only in the nucleus of activated T cells, and a constitutively expressed cytoplasmic component that translocates to the nucleus during T cell activation (Flanagan *et al,* 1991; Jain *et al,* 1991; Boise *et al* 1993; Northrop *et al,* 1993). Part of the calcium signalling requirement for NFAT and hence *IL2* expression is that intracellular $Ca^{2+}i$ regulates the activity of a phosphatase calcineurin, which then controls the translocation of the NFAT cytoplasmic component to the nucleus (Flanagan *et al,* 1991; Clipstone and Crabtree, 1992). $p21^{ras}$ is a synergistic partner with calcineurin for NFAT induction (Woodrow *et al,* 1993a) and is a potent regulator of kinase cascades that activate AP1 protein expression and function (Hunter and Karin, 1992; Karin, 1991).

When the effect of $p21^{v\text{-}Ha\ ras}$ on AP1, NFAT and *IL2* gene induction is compared, the data show that the constitutively active RAS mutant can completely substitute for phorbol esters for AP1 and NFAT induction but is a much poorer substitute in *IL2* gene induction (Rayter *et al,* 1992; Woodrow *et al,* 1993a). These data show that at least three signals are required for *IL2* induction: RAS, calcium and a third signal that is almost certainly provided by PKC (Fig. 1).

## RAS AND PKC REGULATE THE MITOGEN ACTIVATED PROTEIN KINASE SIGNALLING CASCADE DURING T CELL ACTIVATION

In fibroblasts and the phaeochromocytoma PC12 cell line, the transmission of signals from PKC or $p21^{ras}$ to the nucleus appears to involve regulation of the activity of mitogen activated protein (MAP) kinases (Fig. 2) (extracellular signal regulated kinases, ERKs) (Leevers and Marshall, 1992; Pelech and Sanghera, 1992; Robbins *et al,* 1992; Thomas *et al,* 1992). T lymphocytes express at least two MAP kinases, ERK1 and ERK2, that are stimulated in response to TCR triggering (Whitehurst *et al,* 1992). Two intracellular pathways for ERK2 regulation co-exist in T cells: one mediated by RAS, the other by PKC (Izquierdo *et al,* 1993). The TCR stimulates both $p21^{ras}$ and PKC, but data obtained from transfection studies show that expression of the inhibitory RAS mutant $N17^{ras}$, which prevents endogenous RAS activation, suppresses TCR induction of ERK2 (Izquierdo *et al,* 1993). Accordingly, it appears that $p21^{ras}$, and not PKC, couples the TCR to the regulation of MAP kinases. Mitogen activated protein kinases translocate to the nucleus when activated, and their known substrates include transcriptional factors such as Elk1, c-jun and c-myc (Pulverer *et al,* 1991; Seth *et al,* 1992; Marais *et al,* 1993). Thus, one mechanism whereby $p21^{ras}$ could couple the TCR to the nucleus is via stimulation of the ERK kinase cascade (Fig. 2).

The activity of the MAP kinases requires their simultaneous phosphorylation on both tyrosine and threonine (Leevers and Marshall, 1992). The phosphorylation and activation of MAP kinase is induced by an activator kinase, MAP kinase kinase (MAPKK). The link between $p21^{ras}$ and the MAPKK is provided by at least one other kinase (MAPKKK). Two candidates for the MAPKKK have been described, the proto-oncogene Raf-1 (Howe *et al,* 1992) and a kinase termed MEK1 (Lange-Carter *et al,* 1993). Raf-1 can be regulated by at least two pathways: one mediated by $p21^{ras}$ (Howe *et al,* 1992)

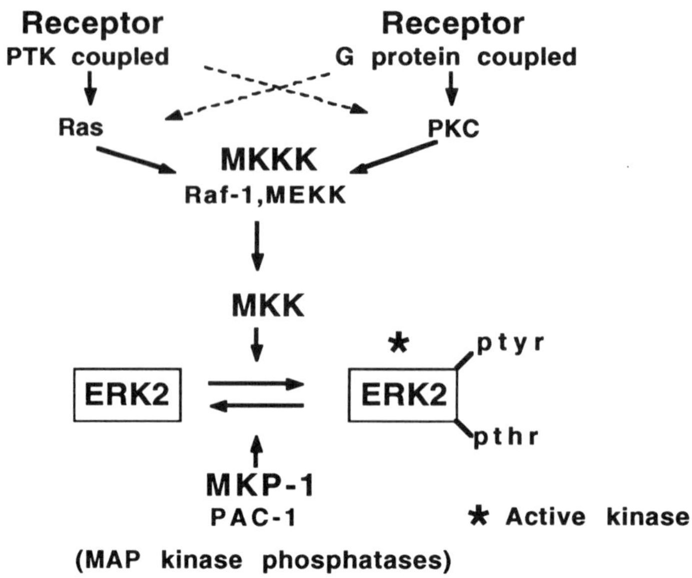


**Fig. 2.** Regulation of MAP kinases. MKKK = MAP kinase kinase kinase, MKP-1 = MAP kinase phosphatase 1

and one controlled by PKC (Sozeri *et al,* 1992). Raf1 is apparently activated in T cells by both TCR and PKC (Siegal *et al,* 1993) and may provide the link between RAS or PKC and ERK2. Accordingly, the positioning of RAS in the mechanisms that couple the TCR and ERK2 provides a framework for positioning other potentially important signalling molecules in the TCR signal transduction pathways. Finally, in vivo phosphorylation levels always reflect the balance of the activities of kinases and phosphatases, and phosphatase activity in the cell may be rate limiting for Raf-1 regulation of ERK2 (Samuels *et al,* 1993). Recent studies have identified a dual specificity phosphatase, MKP1, that dephosphorylates ERK2 in vivo (Sun *et al,* 1993). A related dual specificity phosphatase, PAC1, is expressed in mitogen activated T cells (Rohan *et al,* 1993). It is thus possible that the TCR normally regulates ERK2 by controlling the activities of positive regulators of ERK2 such as $p21^{ras}$ and negative regulators such as PAC1.

## SUMMARY

T cell activation is triggered by antigen stimulation and is characterized by the production of a wide range of cytokines and other immunomodulators crucial for the growth and development of other haemopoietic cells. Activation also induces the T cells to express, on their cell surface, receptors that enable the T cell to respond to the various cytokines generated during an immune response. One well characterized event that occurs when mature T cells are activated is the production of the cytokine IL2 and the acquisition by the T cell of IL2 receptors. Interaction between IL2 and its cellular receptor then directs T cell growth. Expression of the *IL2* gene in T cells is regulated by signalling pathways that originate from the T cell antigen receptor complex (TCR). This review discusses the role of p21$^{ras}$ in these events. The TCR regulates the activity of p21$^{ras}$, and a range of experiments have shown that p21$^{ras}$ couples the TCR to an intracellular kinase cascade involving the serine/threonine kinase Raf-1 and the MAP kinase ERK2. Analysis of more distal receptor signals shows that p21$^{ras}$ controls a signalling pathway that cooperates with a calcium/calcineurin controlled signalling system to stimulate the transcriptional factor NFAT and hence the *IL2* gene. These studies identify p21$^{ras}$ as a critical signalling molecule in immune cells.

## References

Adams JM, Houston H, Allen J, Lints T and Harvey R (1992) The hematopoietically expressed vav proto-oncogene shares homology with the dbl GDP-GTP exchange factor, the bcr gene and a yeast gene (CDC24) involved in cytoskeletal organization. *Oncogene* **7** 611–618

Baldari CT, Macchia G and Telford JL (1992) Interleukin-2 promoter activation in T cells expressing activated Ha-ras. *Journal of Biological Chemistry* **267** 4289–4291

Ballester R, Marchuk D, Boguski M *et al* (1990) The NF1 locus encodes a protein functionally related to mammalian GAP and yeast IRA proteins. *Cell* **63** 851–859

Berridge MJ and Irvine RF (1989) Inositol phosphates and cell signalling. *Nature* **341** 197–205

Berry N and Nishizuka Y (1989) Protein kinase C and T cell activation. *European Journal of Biochemistry* **89** 205–214

Boise LH, Petryniak B, Mao X *et al* (1993) The NFAT-1 DNA binding complex in activated T cells contains Fra-1 and Jun-B. *Molecular and Cellular Biology* **113** 1911–1920

Bowtell D, Fu P, Simon M and Senior P (1992) Identification of murine homologues of the *Drosophila Son of Sevenless* gene:potential activators of ras. *Proceedings of the National Academy of Sciences of the USA* **89** 6511–6515

Buday L and Downward J (1993a) Epidermal growth factor regulates the exchange rate of guanine nucleotides on p21ras in fibroblasts. *Molecular and Cellular Biology* **13** 1903–1910

Buday L and Downward J (1993b) Epidermal growth factor regulates p21ras through the formation of a complex of receptor Grb2 adapter protein and Sos nucleotide exchange factor. *Cell* **73** 611–620

Cantrell DA, Collins MK and Crumpton MJ (1988) Autocrine regulation of T-lymphocyte proliferation: differential induction of IL-2 and IL-2 receptor. *Immunology* **65** 343–349

Clipstone NA and Crabtree GR (1992) Identification of calcineurin as a key signalling enzyme in T-lymphocyte activation. *Nature* **357** 695–697

Crabtree GR (1989) Contingent genetic regulatory events in T lymphocyte activation. *Science* **243** 355–361

Downward J (1992) Regulation of p21ras by GAPs and guanine nucleotide exchange proteins in normal and oncogenic cells. *Current Opinion in Genetics and Development* **2** 13–18

Downward J, Graves JD, Warne PH, Rayter S and Cantrell DA (1990) Stimulation of p21ras upon T-cell activation. *Nature* **346** 719–723

Downward J, Graves JD and Cantrell DA (1992) The regulation and function of p21ras in T lymphocytes. *Immunology Today* **13** 89–92

Durand DB, Bush MR, Morgan JG, Weiss A and Crabtree GR (1987) A 275 basepair fragment at the 5′ end of the interleukin 2 gene enhances expression from a heterologous promoter in response to signals from the T cell antigen receptor. *Journal of Experimental Medicine* **165** 395–407

Egan SE, Giddings BW, Brooks MW, Buday L, Sizeland AM and Weinberg RE (1993) Association of SOS Ras exchange protein with GRB2 is implicated in tyrosine kinase signal transduction and transformation. *Nature* **363** 45–51

Emmel EA, Verweij CL, Durand DB, Higgins KM, Lacy E and Crabtree GR (1989) Cyclosporin A specifically inhibits function of nuclear proteins involved in T cell activation. *Science* **246** 1617–1620

Flanagan WM, Corthesy B, Bram RJ and Crabtree GR (1991) Nuclear association of a T-cell transcription factor blocked by FK-506 and cyclosporin A. *Nature* **352** 803–807

Graves JD, Downward J, Rayter S *et al* (1991) CD2 antigen mediated activation of the guanine nucleotide binding proteins p21ras in human T lymphocytes. *Journal of Immunology* **146** 3709–3712

Gulbins E, Coggeshall KM, Baier G, Katzav S, Burn P and Altman A (1993) Tyrosine kinase stimulated guanine nucleotide exchange of Vav in T cell activation. *Science* **260** 822–825

Howe LR, Leevers SJ, Gomez N, Nakielney S, Cohen P and Marshall CJ (1992) Activation of the MAP kinase pathway by the protein kinase raf. *Cell* **71** 335–342

Hunter T and Karin M (1992) The regulation of transcription by phosphorylation. *Cell* **70** 375–387

Izquierdo M, Downward J, Graves JD and Cantrell DA (1992) Role of protein kinase C in T-cell antigen receptor regulation of p21ras: evidence that two p21ras regulatory pathways coexist in T cells. *Molecular and Cellular Biology* **12** 3305–3312

Izquierdo M, Leevers SJ, Marshall CJ and Cantrell DA (1993) $p21^{ras}$ couples the T cell antigen receptor to extracellular signal-regulated kinase 2 in T lymphocytes. *Journal of Experimental Medicine* **178** 1199–1208

Jain J, McCaffrey PG, Valge-Archer VE and Rao A (1992) Nuclear factor of activated T cells contains Fos and Jun. *Nature* **356** 801–804

Janeway CA and Golstein P (1992) Lymphocyte activation and effector functions. *Current Opinion in Immunology* **4** 265–270

June CH, Fletcher MC, Ledbetter JA *et al* (1990) Inhibition of tyrosine phosphorylation prevents T cell receptor-mediated signal transduction. *Proceedings of the National Academy of Sciences of the USA* **87** 7722–7726

Karin M (1991) Signal transduction and gene control. *Current Opinion in Cell Biology* **3** 467–473

Klausner RD and Samelson LE (1991) T cell antigen receptor activation pathways: the tyrosine kinase connection. *Cell* **64** 875–878

Lange-Carter CA, Pleiman CM, Gardner AM, Blumer KJ and Johnson GL (1993) A divergence in the MAP kinase regulatory network defined by MEK kinase and Raf. *Science* **260** 315–319

Leevers SJ and Marshall CJ (1992) MAP kinase regulation—the oncogene conection. *Trends in Cell Biology* **2** 283–286

McCormick F (1989) ras GTPase activating protein: signal transmitter and signal terminator. *Cell* **56** 5–8

McCormick F (1993) How receptors turn Ras on. *Nature* **363** 15–16

Marais R, Wynne J and Treisman R (1993) The SRF accessory protein ELK-1 contains a growth factor-regulated transcriptional activation domain. *Cell* **73** 381–393

Medema RH, Vries-Smits AMM, van der Zon GCM, Maassen JA and Bos JL (1993) Ras activation by insulin and epidermal growth factor through enhanced exchange of guanine nucleotides on p21ras. *Molecular and Cellular Biology* **13** 155–162

Nishizuka Y (1988) The molecular heterogeneity of protein kinase C and its implication for cellular regulation. *Nature* **334** 661–665

Northrop JP, Ullman KS and Crabtree GR (1993) Characterization of the nuclear and cytoplasmic components of the lymphoid-specific nuclear factor of activated T cells (NFAT) complex. *Journal of Biological Chemistry* **268** 22917–22925

Pelech SL and Sanghera JS (1992) MAP kinases: charting the regulatory pathways. *Science* **257** 1355–1356

Pulverer BJ, Kyriakis JM, Avruch J, Nikolakaki E and Wood gett JR (1991) Phosphorylation of

c-jun mediated by MAP kinases. *Nature* **353** 670
Rayter S, Woodrow M, Lucas SC, Cantrell D and Downward J (1992) p21ras mediates control of IL2 gene promoter function in T cell activation. *EMBO Journal* **11** 4549–4556
Reth M (1989) Antigen receptor tail clue. *Nature* **338** 383–384
Robbins DJ, Cheng M, Zhen E, Vanderbilt CA, Feig LA and Cobb MH (1992) Evidence for a Ras-dependent extracellular signal-regulated protein kinase (ERK) cascade. *Proceedings of the National Academy of Sciences of the USA* **89** 6924–6928
Rohan PJ, Davis P, Moskaluk CA *et al* (1993) Pac-1: a mitogen induced nuclear protein tyrosine phosphatase. *Science* **259** 1763–1766
Samuels ML, Weber MJ, Bishop MJ and McMahon M (1993) Conditional transformation of cells and rapid activation of the mitogen-activated protein kinase cascade by an estradial dependent human Raf-1 protein kinase. *Molecular and Cellular Biology* **13** 6241–6252
Satoh T, Nafakuku M and Kaziro Y (1992) Function of Ras as a molecular switch in signal transduction. *Journal of Biological Chemistry* **267** 24149–24152
Seth A, Gonzalez FA, Gupta S, Radenm DL and Davis RJ (1992) Signal transduction within the nucleus by mitogen-activated protein kinase. *Journal of Biological Chemistry* **34** 24796–24804
Shou C, Farnsworth CL, Neel BG and Feig LA (1992) Molecular cloning of cDNAs encoding a guanine-nucleotide-releasing factor for Ras p21. *Nature* **358** 351–354
Siegal JN, June CH, Yamada H, Rapp U and Samelson LE (1993) Rapid activation of c-Raf-1 after stimulation of the T cell antigen receptor or the muscarinic receptor type 1 in resting T cells. *Journal of Immunology* **151** 4116–4127
Sozeri O, Vollmer K, Liyanage M *et al* (1992) Activation of the c-Raf protein kinase by protein kinase C phosphorylation. *Oncogene* **7** 2259–2262
Sun H, Charles CH, Lau LF and Tonks NK (1993) MKP-1 (3CH134) an immediate early gene product is a dual specificity phosphatase that dephosphorylates MAP kinase in vivo. *Cell* **75** 487–493
Thomas SM, DeMarco M, D'Arcangelo G, Halegoua S and Brugge JS (1992) Ras is essential for nerve growth factor and phorbol ester-induced tyrosine phosphorylation of MAP kinases. *Cell* **68** 1031–1040
Verweij CL, Guidos C and Crabtree GR (1990) Cell type specificity and activation requirements for NFAT-1 (nuclear factor of activated T-cells) transcriptional activity determined by a new method using transgenic mice to assay transcriptional activity of an activated nuclear factor. *Journal of Biological Chemistry* **265** 15788–15795
Weiss A (1993) T cell antigen receptor signal transduction: a tail of tails and cytoplasmic protein-tyrosine kinases. *Cell* **73** 209–212
Weiss A and Imboden JB (1987) Cell surface molecules and early events involved in human T lymphocyte activation. *Advances in Immunology* **41** 1–38
Weiss A, Koretzky G, Schatzmann RC and Kadlecec T (1991) Functional activation of the T cell antigen receptor induces tyrosine phosphorylation of phospholipase C gamma1. *Proceedings of the National Academy of Sciences of the USA* **88** 5484–5488
Weissman AM, Bonifacino JS, Klausner RD, Samelson LE and O'Shea JJ (1989) T cell antigen receptor: structure assembly and function. *Year Immunology* **4** 74–93
Whitehurst CE, Boulton TG, Cobb MH and Geppert TG (1992) Extracellular signal-regulated kinases in T cells: anti-CD3 and 4beta-phorbol 12-myristate 13-acetate-induced phosphorylation and activation. *Journal of Immunology* **148** 3230–3237
Woodrow M, Clipstone N and Cantrell DA (1993a) p21ras and calcineurin synergize to regulate NFAT. *Journal of Experimental Medicine* **178** 1517–1522
Woodrow M, Rayter S, Downward J and Cantrell DA (1993b) p21ras function is important for T cell antigen receptor and protein kinase C regulation of nuclear factor of activated cells. *Journal of Immunology* **150** 1–9

The authors are responsible for the accuracy of the references.

# Control of T Cell Development by Non-receptor Protein Tyrosine Kinases

**ROGER M PERLMUTTER**

*Howard Hughes Medical Institute and Departments of Immunology, Biochemistry and Medicine, University of Washington, Seattle, WA 98915*



## INTRODUCTION

Virtually all circulating T lymphocytes arise from haemopoietic progenitors that mature within the thymus (von Boehmer, 1988). T cells themselves are principally responsible for the self/non-self discrimination that is the hallmark of adaptive immunity. As such, the mechanism whereby populations of such cells become insensitive (tolerant) to host proteins while retaining the ability to respond vigorously to foreign polypeptides is of fundamental importance. During the past few years, it has become apparent that individual antigen receptors on the surfaces of T lymphocytes can, depending on the circumstances, deliver very different signals to the cell interior. For example, T lymphocytes, upon encountering an antigen, may proliferate ("activation"), may become refractory to subsequent stimulation ("anergy") or may actually undergo programmed cell death ("apoptosis"), all in response to signals delivered from a single type of antigen receptor (Schwartz, 1989).

To make sense of antigen recognition by T cells, a more comprehensive understanding of the signalling process that links the T cell antigen receptor to these heterogeneous outcomes must be achieved. This is nowhere more apparent than in the process of T cell development, where signals from the T cell antigen receptor permit selective pruning of thymocyte populations such that self reactive cells are largely eliminated while thymocytes bearing receptors that represent appropriate specificities are released into the circulation. In the following pages, I describe aspects of the biochemistry of T cell receptor sig-

*Cancer Surveys* Volume 22: *Molecular Mechanisms of the Immune Response*

nalling, focusing on a set of non-receptor protein tyrosine kinases that participate in the regulation of all T cell responses. In particular, I review recent studies demonstrating that $p56^{lck}$, a lymphocyte specific membrane associated protein tyrosine kinase, is a crucial regulator of T cell receptor gene rearrangement and of thymopoiesis in general. This analysis is offered as a tribute to Dr Michael J Crumpton, whose broad interests in protein structure and in immune function led him to characterize important aspects of lymphocyte signalling responses.

## FUNDAMENTALS OF THYMOCYTE MATURATION

In the mouse, the initial colonization of the thymus during fetal ontogeny appears to occur in waves, such that early stem cells (those that arrive before to day 16 of gestation) give rise to progeny that express T cell receptor heterodimers of the γ/δ type, whereas the progenitors that populate the thymus subsequently generate primarily cells of the more familiar type that express α/β T cell receptors (Raulet *et al,* 1991). Studies of T cell receptor gene rearrangements have yielded data most consistent with the view that T cells bearing γ/δ receptors arise from a lineage that is independent of that which generates α/β cells (Winoto and Baltimore, 1989). Considering thymopoiesis generally, as it occurs from fetal day 17 until thymic involution supervenes in the sexually mature adult, two principal events take place. Firstly, rapid cell divisions permit the generation of large numbers of T lymphocytes (about $10^8$/day by most estimates) from a small population of immature progenitors; and secondly, a form of cellular redaction must occur to permit the selective export of cells that recognize foreign peptide antigens in the context of self MHC molecules but which are not autoreactive. This moulding of the T cell repertoire itself reflects two different kinds of selection events: recruitment of cells bearing functional antigen receptors (positive selection) and elimination of self reactive cells (negative selection).

Although the molecular events underlying thymocyte maturation are necessarily complex, a fairly precise description of cell populations that represent intermediate states of maturity can be achieved by simply examining the expression of the T cell receptor (usually carried out with antibodies directed against the CD3 ε polypeptide) and the CD4 and CD8 co-receptors. Immature thymocytes, representing approximately 2% of total cells, lack expression of all three markers. These cells give rise to a population that expresses both CD4 and CD8 simultaneously (nearly 85% of cells), which in turn gives rise to cells that express either CD4 or CD8 molecules in a mutually exclusive fashion. Within the $CD4^+8^+$ precursor population, about half of the cells express the antigen receptor (usually at fairly low levels). These cells serve as the substrate for positive and negative selection events that ensure elimination of dysfunctional or self reactive T cells, yielding $CD4^+8^-$ or $CD4^-8^+$ cells that recognize antigen in association with class II or class I antigen presentation molecules, respectively. These "single positive" cells, poised to leave the thymus, are the immediate precursors of mature circulating T cells and express high levels of the T cell antigen receptor (von Boehmer, 1988).

Virtually all cell divisions in the thymus occur before the $CD4^{+}8^{+}$ stage, in a small population of immature $CD4^{-}8^{-}$ or $CD4^{-}8^{lo}$ thymoblasts. In addition to the increase in mean cell volume that accompanies entry into a proliferative state, a set of other cell surface markers can be used to define developmental waypoints in the thymocyte maturation sequence. For example, $CD4^{-}8^{-}$ cells initially express the interleukin 2 (IL2) receptor α chain, and then become $IL2R^{-}$, at which point cell division proceeds. Figure 1 provides a schematic diagram outlining the stages of thymocyte maturation. The process whereby functional T cell receptor α and β genes are assembled from widely dispersed gene segments is also developmentally ordered in thymocytes, with β chain gene rearrangements confined primarily to $CD4^{-}8^{-}$ cells that bear the IL2 receptor, and α chain gene rearrangements occurring subsequently. As described below, considerable evidence supports the view that creation of a functional T cell receptor β chain transcriptional unit provides a signal that permits the maturation process to proceed.

## INVOLVEMENT OF THE T CELL RECEPTOR IN REGULATING T CELL DEVELOPMENT

Moulding of the T cell receptor repertoire by elimination of unsuitable thymocytes requires that each cell expresses only a single type of antigen receptor binding site. For T cell receptors, as for analogous surface antibodies on B lymphocytes, this is achieved through a process of allelic exclusion, wherein the receptor is encoded by only one of two allelic gene sets. More precisely, each T cell receptor gene is assembled from gene segments, positioned discontinuously in germline DNA, that are juxtaposed by site specific and developmentally regulated gene rearrangement events during thymopoiesis (Kronenberg *et al,* 1986). Initially, T cell receptor β chain gene rearrangements occur, linking a D gene segment with a J gene segment and thereafter a V gene segment with the DJ unit. The α locus rearranges subsequently, permitting juxtaposition of a V gene segment with a J gene segment. In general, although joining of $D_{\beta}$ to $J_{\beta}$ may occur on both chromosome homologues, a functional $V_{\beta}$ gene segment rearrangement occurs on only a single allele. Regulated catalysis of $V_{\alpha}$ to $J_{\alpha}$ rearrangements also occurs, but significantly more violations of strict allelic exclusion are observed at this locus. In principle, two alternative mechanisms could be invoked to explain allelic exclusion. Firstly, if the probability of generating a functional rearrangement is sufficiently low, simple stochastic processes could assure that few cells would emerge with productive rearrangements on both β (or α) encoding homologues. Alternatively, productive assembly of a β chain transcriptional

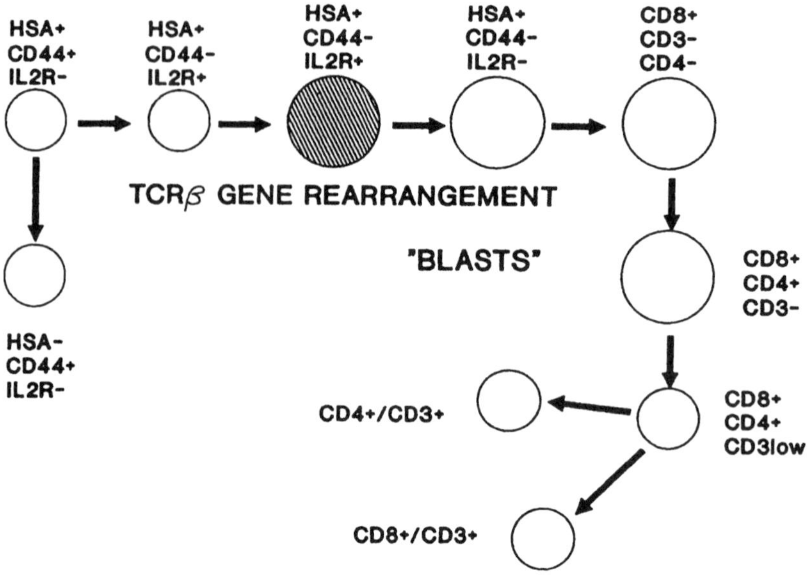


**Fig. 1.** Features of early thymocyte development. Cell populations are represented by circles. The cell surface phenotype of each population is noted. Arrows denote the direction of the maturation sequence. Larger circles indicate cells with blast characteristics. The shaded circle denotes the point where expression of T cell receptor β chain (TCRβ) is required for subsequent development. Adapted from Levin *et al* (1993)

unit could send a signal that would arrest subsequent rearrangements at the β locus. Most evidence supports the latter view. For example, introduction of a functionally rearranged β chain transgene blocks endogenous $V_\beta$ gene rearrangement almost completely (von Boehmer, 1990). Since many cells can be found that contain both a functional β chain gene rearrangement and an out of frame rearrangement on the opposite allele (Kronenberg *et al,* 1986), it appears that generation of a satisfactory β chain reading frame is required to permit operation of the signalling mechanism that controls allelic exclusion. Other experiments in transgenic mice indicate that synthesis of a truncated β chain, including only the transmembrane region and the intracytoplasmic tail (the latter representing just six aminoacid residues), blocks endogenous rearrangements effectively (Krimpenfort *et al,* 1989).

The importance of β chain derived signals in thymocyte maturation can be further appreciated by examining the characteristics of mice bearing a targeted mutation of the β locus (Mombaerts *et al,* 1992). Thymocyte maturation in such mice fails almost completely, leaving primarily $CD4^-8^-$ cells that do not progress beyond the IL2 receptor bearing stage. The same phenotype obtains in mice lacking either the *RAG1* or *RAG2* gene, both of which are required for normal rearrangement. However, in such mice, the developmental disturbance can be ameliorated by introduction of a functional T cell receptor β chain transgene (Shinkai *et al,* 1993). These observations demonstrate that signals provoked by synthesis of the T cell receptor β chain instruct developing

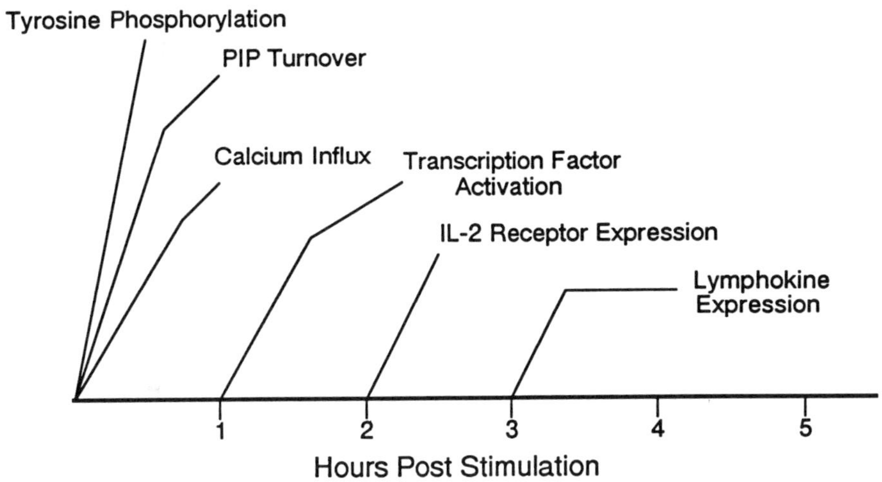


**Fig. 2.** Key biochemical events associated with T cell activation. A set of readily measured biochemical changes that occur following ligand occupancy of the T cell receptor is oriented along an x axis time line. PIP = phosphatidylinositol-bis-phosphate

thymocytes to stop further β chain gene rearrangement and to continue maturation, in part by permitting rearrangement of the T cell receptor α locus and by driving both proliferation and the expression of the CD4 and CD8 co-receptors (Mombaerts *et al,* 1992).

In addition to sending these signals promoting thymocyte maturation, the T cell receptor heterodimer, along with its CD3 components and the CD4 and CD8 co-receptors, delivers the signals that trigger cell death versus survival in the moulding of the T cell receptor repertoire (von Boehmer, 1988, 1990). Thus, it is reasonable to inquire whether the signalling mechanisms that permit β chain driven thymocyte maturation and subsequent T cell repertoire selection utilize the same molecular elements. Insights into this process have emerged from study of the biochemistry of T cell signalling.

## BIOCHEMISTRY OF SIGNALLING FROM THE T CELL RECEPTOR

### Metabolic Events following T Cell Receptor Stimulation

Ligand occupancy of the T cell receptor provokes a stereotyped series of biochemical responses beginning with the accumulation of substrates phosphorylated on tyrosine, the subsequent turnover of membrane phospholipids and mobilization of intracellular calcium stores and ultimately the activation of transcription factors that promote the expression of cytokines and their receptors (Fig. 2) (Perlmutter *et al,* 1993). In light of the apparently contingent nature of these events, attention has focused on the protein tyrosine kinases and phosphotyrosine phosphatases that act in T lymphocytes. For example, T cell activation can be blocked almost completely at its earliest stages by relatively non-selective protein tyrosine kinase inhibitors (Mustelin *et al,* 1990). In addition, mutant T cells lacking the CD45 phosphotyrosine phosphatase fail to respond to T cell receptor stimulation (Pingel and Thomas, 1989).

### Non-receptor Protein Tyrosine Kinases

Among those protein tyrosine kinases that might serve to link the T cell receptor to the cell interior, two SRC family molecules, $p59^{fyn}$ and $p56^{lck}$, have attracted special interest. The *FYN* gene encodes a 532 aminoacid polypeptide that is expressed primarily in neuronal cells and in T lymphocytes. The gene itself contains two alternative exons 7, and as a result of mutually exclusive alternative splicing, exon 7A is preferentially incorporated into transcripts that accumulate in neurons, whereas exon 7B contributes to those transcripts that accumulate in T cells (Cooke and Perlmutter, 1989). Data supporting the role of $p59^{fyn}$ in T cell receptor signalling derive largely from the study of mouse mutants in which *FYN* expression has been manipulated. Thus, thymocyte specific overexpression of $p59^{fyn}$ in transgenic mice yields cells that respond more vigorously than do normal cells when exposed to a T cell receptor specific stimulus (Cooke *et al,* 1991). By contrast, the thymocytes of mice bearing a targeted disruption of the *FYN* gene (and hence lacking expression of $p59^{fyn}$) appear to develop normally but manifest a dramatic reduction in the ability to transmit T cell receptor derived signals in mature $CD4^{+}8^{-}$ or $CD4^{-}8^{+}$ cells (Appleby *et al,* 1992; Stein *et al,* 1992). Expression of $p59^{fyn}$ is ordinarily confined to mature thymocyte subpopulations (Cooke *et al,* 1991). These data permit two important conclusions: $p59^{fyn}$ participates in relaying signals from the antigen receptor in at least some T lineage cells, and the regulation of early thymocyte development by the T cell receptor β chain cannot be mediated by $p59^{fyn}$ (since this kinase is not normally expressed in these immature cells and disruption of the *FYN* gene does not compromise thymocyte development). Hence, some other molecule must relay signals that permit allelic exclusion at the T cell receptor β locus. Considerable evidence supports the view that $p56^{lck}$ serves this function.

## INVOLVEMENT OF $p56^{lck}$ IN CONTROLLING THYMOCYTE MATURATION

Insight into the importance of $p56^{lck}$ in the control of thymocyte development came first from the study of mice bearing *LCK* transgenes. Transcripts from the *LCK* locus accumulate in all normal T lineage cells, so far as is known, and in NK cells and some B cells as well (Marth *et al,* 1985). Two distinct promoters direct *LCK* transcription: a 3′(proximal) promoter drives the accumulation of transcripts in all thymocyte populations but especially in immature cells, and a 5′(distal) promoter acts in mature circulating T cells (Wildin *et al,* 1991). The *LCK* gene is expressed at highest levels in immature thymocytes, reflecting the activity of the proximal promoter. Remarkably, augmented expression of wild type *LCK* transcripts, achieved with an *LCK* minigene in transgenic mice, yielded cells in which rearrangement of $V_\beta$ gene segments was specifically interdicted (Abraham *et al,* 1991a; Anderson *et al,* 1992). Mice carrying this transgene produced normal numbers of thymocytes, but their cells failed to express the T cell receptor complex because functional $\beta$ chains were not synthesized. This defect could be completely reversed by artificial provision of a functionally rearranged transgenic T cell receptor $\beta$ chain gene (Anderson *et al,* 1992). Thus, cells in which $p56^{lck}$ activity was augmented behaved as if they were responding to the signal that ordinarily results from expression of a T cell receptor $\beta$ chain.

Experiments in which *LCK* function was compromised proved even more revealing. For example, mice lacking $p56^{lck}$ as a result of targeted disruption of the *LCK* locus contained very few thymocytes, most of which lacked both CD4 and CD8 expression (Molina *et al,* 1992). This phenotype resembles that observed following targeted disruption of the T cell receptor $\beta$ locus itself (Mombaerts *et al,* 1992). Additional insight into this phenomenon derived from analysis of mice expressing high levels of a dominant negative *LCK* transgene encoding a catalytically inactive form of $p56^{lck}$. By examining a large number of different mouse lines, it was possible to establish a dose-response curve for the effects of this transgene (Levin *et al,* 1993). A simple first order exponential relationship describes the effect of increasing ratios of active to inactive $p56^{lck}$ kinase on the number of thymocytes and on their development. Animals expressing a 12-fold excess of catalytically inactive $p56^{lck}$ have thymuses that contain only 2% the normal number of cells, and all of the residual thymocytes in such animals are $CD4^-8^-$ $G_1$ blasts bearing high levels of the IL2 receptor $\alpha$ chain. Thus, interference with $p56^{lck}$ function appears to block thymocyte development in precisely the way that would be expected if this kinase ordinarily acts to signal production of a T cell receptor $\beta$ chain during thymocyte development. Moreover, in its simplest form, the exponential relationship between $p56^{lck}$ function and thymocyte development suggests that mitogenesis in immature thymoblasts requires $p56^{lck}$ and that seven symmetrical cell divisions separate immature $CD4^-8^-$ cells from the resting $CD4^+8^+$ cells to which they give rise (Levin *et al,* 1993). In this light, it is intriguing that very high level expression of $p56^{lck}$ in transgenic mice leads to the development of aggressive thymic tumours consisting exclusively of immature cells (Abraham *et al,* 1991b).

The hypothesis that $p56^{lck}$ serves as the sensing mechanism that signals synthesis of a T cell receptor $\beta$ chain makes two very strong predictions. Firstly, this hypothesis demands that interference with $p56^{lck}$ function will lead to violation of allelic exclusion at the $\beta$ locus. A simple test of this prediction was established by introducing a functional T cell receptor $\beta$ chain transgene into mice bearing the dominant negative *LCK* constructs. In three separate lines of such doubly transgenic animals, the presence of the $\beta$ transgene was no longer sufficient to block rearrangement of endogenous $V_\beta$ gene segments (Anderson *et al,* 1993). This unprecedented violation of allelic exclusion argues strongly

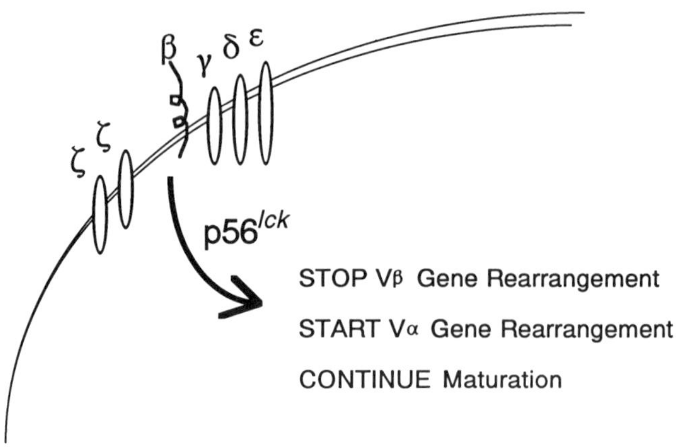


**Fig. 3.** Involvement of p56$^{lck}$ in regulating thymocyte developmnent. See text for details

that p56$^{lck}$ function is required for satisfactory ordering of T cell receptor gene rearrangements during thymocyte development.

A second prediction of the model linking p56$^{lck}$ function to T cell receptor β chain signalling is that the compromise in thymocyte development resulting from congenital absence of a functional T cell receptor β chain could be largely reversed if an adventitious p56$^{lck}$ signal could instead be provided. This prediction has also been verified in transgenic model systems (Anderson SJ and Perlmutter RM, unpublished results).

Together, these data are in accord with a model outlined in Fig. 3, in which p56$^{lck}$ would act during thymocyte development to sense the synthesis of a T cell receptor β chain and to promote $V_\alpha$ rearrangement, suppress further $V_\beta$ rearrangement and stimulate maturation. This model leaves undescribed the nature of the molecular structure with which p56$^{lck}$ interacts to sense β chain synthesis. For example, although a surface receptor complex including the β chain might serve this function, other alternative models, including some that postulate sequestration of p56$^{lck}$ via a β chain inhibitable process, can easily be generated. The model also fails to provide any specific information about the mechanism whereby p56$^{lck}$, once activated, delivers its specialized signal. Elucidation of the chain of molecular events linking p56$^{lck}$ to the nucleus will provide important new insights into the control of thymocyte development.

## SPECULATIONS ON THE IMPORTANCE OF OTHER SIGNALLING MOLECULES

Experiments using whole animal model systems have provided considerable insight into the mechanisms whereby T cell receptor signals are interpreted in thymocytes. However, a fundamental problem remains: ligand occupancy of the antigen receptor can provoke very different responses depending on the nature of the stimulating event. In the case of thymocyte selection, two contrasting outcomes (recruitment vs apoptotic death) can result from stimulation of individual T cell receptors. To date, no biochemical distinctions have been made in the signalling pathways that emanate from the antigen receptor under these circumstances. However, as regards selection itself, there is good reason to believe that $p59^{fyn}$, an important contributor to proliferative responses in mature thymocytes and T cells, has no role. The importance of $p56^{lck}$ is more difficult to assess, since alterations in its function affect earlier events in thymocyte development. However, and precisely for this reason, it is apparent that even if $p56^{lck}$ is required for positive selection, additional signalling molecules must modify its effects at this later stage in the maturation sequence. This reasoning has encouraged attempts to identify other protein tyrosine kinases that might assist in regulating thymocyte selection. The *ZAP70* and *SYK* encoded kinases are especially attractive in this regard, since they have been shown to signal effectively in T cells when included in chimaeric transmembrane molecules that bear a CD16 extracellular domain (Kolanus *et al,* 1993). Whether these kinases act in concert with $p56^{lck}$ and $p59^{fyn}$ or independently remains open to question. In either case, protein tyrosine kinase activation must stimulate a set of downstream effector molecules, leading ultimately to changes in the transcription of genes encoding cell surface molecules and lymphokines. The information available from study of $p56^{lck}$ and $p59^{fyn}$ suggests that each protein tyrosine kinase will deliver distinct, non-overlapping signals. Thus, just as $p56^{lck}$ regulates early thymocyte development, whereas $p59^{fyn}$ controls T cell receptor induced proliferative responses in mature cells, the functions of the *ZAP70* and *SYK* encoded kinases should be easy to differentiate. Once this information is in hand, it should be possible to assign other metabolic regulatory circuits to pathways involving one or more of the kinases that co-ordinate early responses. Building upon this knowledge, a complete dissection of the wiring diagram that underlies T cell responsiveness seems achievable.

## SUMMARY

Stimulation of the T cell antigen receptor leads to several possible outcomes. This is especially true in thymocytes, where ligand occupancy of the receptor may promote survival or provoke cell death. Insight into the circuitry of T cell receptor signalling has been achieved in transgenic mouse model systems. In particular, two SRC-family protein tyrosine kinases, $p59^{fyn}$ and $p56^{lck}$, have been shown to participate in controlling mature thymocyte proliferation and immature thymocyte development, respectively. Analysis of the function of $p56^{lck}$ has been especially instructive and has yielded data consistent with a model in which this kinase serves as the gatekeeper at a developmental checkpoint wherein T cell receptor $\beta$ chain synthesis promotes maturation and cell division. In addition, a remarkably coherent data set supports the view that p56[lck] regulates allelic exclusion at the T cell receptor β locus. Further testing of putative signalling molecules in transgenic mice promises to permit elucidation of the biochemical distinctions between positively and negatively selecting stimulation pathways active during T cell development.

## References

Abraham KM, Levin SD, Marth JD, Forbush KA and Perlmutter RM (1991a) Delayed thymocyte development induced by augmented expression of $p56^{lck}$. *Journal of Experimental Medicine* **173** 1421–1432

Abraham KM, Levin SD, Marth JD, Forbush KA and Perlmutter RM (1991b) Thymic tumorigenesis induced by overexpression of $p56^{lck}$. *Proceedings of the National Academy of Sciences of the USA* **88** 3977–3981

Anderson SJ, Abraham KM, Nakayama T, Singer A and Perlmutter RM (1992) Inhibition of T-cell receptor beta-chain gene rearrangement by overexpression of the non-receptor protein tyrosine kinase $p56^{lck}$. *EMBO Journal* **11** 4877–4886

Anderson SJ, Levin SD and Perlmutter RM (1993) The protein tyrosine kinase $p56^{lck}$ controls allelic exclusion of T cell receptor beta chain genes. *Nature* **365** 552–554

Appleby MW, Gross JA, Cooke MP, Levin SD, Qian X and Perlmutter RM (1992) Defective T cell receptor signaling in mice lacking the thymic isoform of $p59^{fyn}$. *Cell* **70** 751–763

Cooke MP and Perlmutter RM (1989) Exclusive expression of a novel form of the *fyn* protooncogene in hematopoietic cells. *New Biologist* **1** 66–74

Cooke MP, Abraham KM, Forbush KA and Perlmutter RM (1991) Regulation of T cell receptor signalling by a *src* family protein-tyrosine kinase ($p59^{fyn}$). *Cell* **65** 281–291

Kolanus W, Romeo C and Seed B (1993) T cell activation by clustered tyrosine kinases. *Cell* **74** 171–183

Krimpenfort P, Ossendorp F, Borst J, Melief C and Berns A (1989) T cell depletion in transgenic mice carrying a mutant gene for TCR-beta. *Nature* **341** 742–746

Kronenberg M, Siu G and Hood LE (1986) The molecular genetics of the T-cell antigen receptor and T-cell antigen recognition. *Annual Review of Immunology* **4** 529–591

Levin SD, Anderson SJ, Forbush KA and Perlmutter RM (1993) A dominant-negative transgene defines a role for $p56^{lck}$ in thymopoiesis. *EMBO Journal* **4** 1671–1680

Marth JD, Peet R, Krebs EG and Perlmutter RM (1985) A lymphocyte-specific protein-tyrosine kinase is rearranged and overexpressed in the murine T cell lymphoma LSTRA. *Cell* **43** 393–404

Molina TJ, Kishihara K, Siderovski DP *et al* (1992) Profound block in thymocyte development in mice lacking $p56^{lck}$. *Nature* **357** 161–164

Mombaerts P, Clarke AR, Rudnicki MA *et al* (1992) Mutations in the T-cell antigen receptor genes alpha and beta block thymocyte development at different stages. *Nature* **360** 225–231

Mustelin T, Coggeshall KM, Isakov N and Altman A (1990) T cell antigen receptor-mediated activation of phospholipase C requires tyrosine phosphorylation. *Science* **247** 1584–1587

Perlmutter RM, Levin SD, Appleby MW, Anderson SJ and Alberola-Ila J (1993) Regulation of lymphocyte function by protein phosphorylation. *Annual Review of Immunology* **11** 451–499

Pingel JT and Thomas ML (1989) Evidence that the leukocyte-common antigen is required for antigen-induced T lymphocyte proliferation. *Cell* **58** 1055–1065

Raulet DH, Spencer DM, Hsiang Y-H *et al* (1991) Control of gamma delta T-cell development. *Immunological Reviews* **120** 185–204

Schwartz RH (1989) Acquistion of immunologic self-tolerance. *Cell* **57** 1073–1081
Shinkai Y, Koyasu S, Nakayama K-I *et al* (1993) Restoration of T cell development in RAG-2-deficient mice by functional TCR transgenes. *Science* **259** 822–825
Stein PL, Lee H-M, Rich S and Soriano P (1992) pp59$^{fyn}$ mutant mice display differential signalling in thymocytes and peripheral T cells. *Cell* **70** 741–750
von Boehmer H (1988) The developmental biology of T lymphocytes. *Annual Review of Immunology* **6** 309–326
von Boehmer H (1990) Developmental biology of T cells in T cell-receptor transgenic mice. *Annual Review of Immunology* **8** 531–556
Wildin RS, Garvin AM, Pawar S *et al* (1991) Developmental regulation of *lck* gene expression in T lymphocytes. *Journal of Experimental Medicine* **173** 383–393
Winoto A and Baltimore D (1989) Separate lineages of T cells expressing the alpha beta and gamma delta receptors. *Nature* **338** 430–432

The author is responsible for the accuracy of the references.

# T Lymphocyte Activation: The Role of Tyrosine Phosphorylation

**DAVID I JACKSON[1] • WINSTON VERBI[1] • ANDREW I LAZAROVITS[2] MICHAEL J CRUMPTON[3]**

*[1]ICRF Applied Development Laboratory, Dominion House, St Bartholomew's Hospital, London EC1A 7BE; [2]University Hospital, Nephrology, 339 Windermere Road, P O Box 5339, London, Ontario N6A 5A5, Canada; [3]Imperial Cancer Research Technology Ltd, Sardinia House, Sardinia Street, London WC2 3NL*



## INTRODUCTION

Engagement of the T cell receptor by antigenic peptide presented by the class II antigens of the major histocompatibility complex (MHC) on the surface of the antigen presenting cell, or by cross linkage of the T cell receptor by homologous antibodies, results in the initiation of activation of several intracellular signalling pathways that ultimately lead to T cell growth and differentiation. The T cell receptor consists of the products of six genes, namely the variable α and β subunits that are non-covalently associated with the invariant chains of the CD3 complex (γ, δ, ε) plus the ζ chains (Clevers *et al,* 1988). Whereas the function of the αβ heterodimer is antigen recognition, the CD3 and ζ polypeptides function primarily as signal transducers, coupling the T cell receptor to downstream signalling pathways. Thus, analyses of genetically engineered chimaeric polypeptides containing the cytoplasmic domains of ε and ζ chains have characterized a sequence motif that is responsible for their signal transducing capability (Weiss, 1993).

Activation via the T cell receptor induces multiple intracellular responses, of which the earliest appears to be the activation of protein tyrosine kinases (PTKs), resulting in the phosphorylation of a host of polypeptides on tyrosine (Ley *et al,* 1991; Samelson and Klausner, 1993). Unlike some other cell surface receptors, such as those for epidermal growth factor or insulin, the T cell receptor apparently does not possess intrinsic kinase activity. Rather, it appears that the cytoplasmic domains of the CD3 and ζ chains are associated directly or indirectly with the src family kinase $p59^{fyn}$ and a novel T cell specific PTK, ZAP70 (Weiss, 1993). The T cell receptor coupled PTKs have an obligate role in regulating the increase in intracellular $[Ca^{++}]$ and the stimulation of protein kinase C, which are consequent to antigen recognition and which make important contributions to the overall process of cell activation (Weiss *et al,* 1991). A second essential PTK regulated pathway links the T cell receptor to the ras guanine nucleotide binding cycle (Downward *et al,* 1992).

Antigen recognition by the T cell receptor incorporates the CD4 (CD8) antigen, whose extracellular domain interacts with the MHC class II (class I) antigen of the antigen presenting cell (Bierer *et al,* 1989). This interaction contributes to the T cell signal response pathway(s) through the non-covalent association of the src family kinase $p56^{lck}$ with the cytoplasmic portion of the CD4 (CD8) antigen (Veillette and Davidson, 1993). Thus, T cells expressing mutant CD4 (CD8) antigens unable to bind $p56^{lck}$ show a much reduced response to antigen recognition. Furthermore, various results indicate that $p56^{lck}$ contributes to, as well as regulates, T cell receptor mediated signalling, a consequence that is not at all surprising given the close physical apposition of the T cell receptor complex with CD4 (CD8) and the physiological requirement for both the T cell receptor and CD4 (CD8) antigen to interact with the antigenic peptide class II (class I) complex.

Although, experimentally, T cell activation is usually achieved by direct targeting of the T cell receptor complex, it can also be induced through the cross linkage of various cell surface molecules either alone or in combination one with another; these molecules include the CD2 (Boyer *et al,* 1993), CD5 (Spertini *et al,* 1991), CD7, CD28 and CD45 antigens. Activation via the latter antigens may reflect their physiological roles as accessory molecules to the T cell receptor in antigen recognition and/or the initiators of alternative signalling response pathways. In common with other cell types, T cell activation initiated via various distinct cell surface "receptors" results in the induction of multiple signal transduction pathways. Comprehension of the specific roles of the individual pathways as well as the probable redundancy and/or cross talk between the different pathways represents a profound challenge.

## PROTEIN TYROSINE KINASES AND T LYMPHOCYTE ACTIVATION

Induction of phosphorylation on tyrosine is clearly crucial to the establishment of the cascade of intracellular biochemical responses following antigen recognition. Although an exact molecular description of the initiating steps of the activation pathway(s) is lacking at present, it is possible to provide a satisfying outline. Given the intimate association of the PTKs $p59^{fyn}$ and $p56^{lck}$ with the T cell receptor and CD4 (CD8) antigen, respectively, of the antigenic peptide class II (I) recognition complex, activation of these kinases is the most probable initiating step. The immediate substrates for tyrosine phosphorylation include phospholipases $C\gamma_1$ and $C\gamma_2$ resulting in their activation and the consequent hydrolysis of phosphatidylinositol ($PIP_2$), which in turn is responsible for the increase in intracellular [$Ca^{++}$] and protein kinase C activation characteristic of T cell receptor complex mediated signalling responses.

Structural studies of the $p56^{lck}$ and $p59^{fyn}$ kinases suggest that they are present in resting cells in an inactive state which depends on their being phosphorylated on tyrosine; and that dephosphorylation is coupled with a conformational change, resulting in the exposure of the kinase domain in an active state (Eck *et al,* 1994). Assuming that this explanation is correct, then the initiation of activation corresponds to a dephosphorylation, that is, the activation of a tyrosine phosphatase. CD45 represents the most compelling candidate for this phosphatase (McFarland *et al,* 1993), a view that is compatible with the demonstration that expression of CD45 is a prerequisite for generating a productive response via the T cell receptor complex (Weiss, 1993). The signal for CD45 activation is not clear, although the observation that its phosphorylation on tyrosine by $p50^{csk}$ kinase creates a binding site for $p56^{lck}$ and that $p56^{lck}$ binding is concomitant with increased phosphatase activity provides a plausible route (Autero *et al,* 1994). A transient association of activated CD45 with the T cell receptor that is promoted by antigen recognition is one direct mechanism by which its activation could be coupled with recognition of antigen.

The above outline of the T cell receptor–CD3 complex initiated signalling response is reasonably satisfying, but undoubtedly it is oversimplistic and fails to incorporate in an integrated way all of the reported data, some of which are currently confusing and apparently contradictory. An especially important question concerns the relative contributions made by $p59^{fyn}$ and $p56^{lck}$ kinases to the response pathway(s). Although activation of $p59^{fyn}$ by cross linkage of the T cell receptor–CD3 complex induces tyrosine phosphorylation of a different set of polypeptides compared with $p56^{lck}$ activation by CD4 (CD8) cross linkage (Veillette *et al,* 1989; Luo and Sefton, 1990), this distinction is unlikely to be important physiologically, because the T cell receptor is coupled directly with CD4 (CD8). One complicating feature may be due to the multiple associations of kinases with cell surface components, which could provide a rational explanation for the ability to initiate T cell activation via multiple surface antigens. Thus, $p59^{fyn}$ is not associated exclusively with the T cell receptor, as illustrated by the murine T cell clone D10, where it has been shown to be linked to a GPI anchored cell surface antigen, Ly-6A, in a manner independent of any T cell receptor association (Lee *et al,* 1994). $p56^{lck}$ kinase activity stimulated by cross linking CD34 apparently has a limited role in T cell activation (Collins and Burakoff, 1993), but this direct interpretation is most probably too superficial and fails to take account of "cross talk" between the kinases, including negative regulation. For example, in D10 cells transfected with antisense $p59^{fyn}$, the reduction in amount of $p59^{fyn}$ was coupled with a decrease in the in vitro $p56^{lck}$ activity; however, normal levels of $p56^{lck}$ protein were detected, leading to the suggestion that $p59^{fyn}$ regulates $p56^{lck}$ in a temporal manner during T cell activation (Lee *et al,* 1994). A similar avenue of regulation of the T cell receptor–CD3 complex associated tyrosine kinase ZAP70 by $p56^{lck}$ has been proposed by Iwashima *et al* (1994).

## SH2 AND SH3 DOMAINS

Tyrosine phosphorylation/dephosphorylation is converted into a propagated signal response through transient specific molecular associations, in which SRC homology 2 (SH2) and 3 (SH3) domains play a most important part (Anderson *et al,* 1990; Songyang *et al,* 1993). SH2 domains possess conserved residues, which form the phosphotyrosine binding pocket, as well as adjacent more variable residues that determine the specificity and affinity of binding, giving rise to a mechanism for recognizing different phosphotyrosine containing peptides (Waksman *et al,* 1992; Songyang *et al,* 1993; Marengere *et al,* 1994). Many intracellular targets of protein tyrosine kinases possess SH2 domains that recognize directly phosphotyrosine containing sites on autophosphorylated kinases and/or their substrates, allowing a complex cascade of interactions to occur during the activation process.

In particular, apart from possessing SH2 domains, $p56^{lck}$ and $p59^{fyn}$ become autophosphorylated on tyrosine, providing a site that is recognized by self SH2 domains, thereby providing a complex web regulating both kinase activity and a cascade of molecular interactions (Sieh *et al,* 1993).

The situation is further complicated by the presence in $p59^{fyn}$ of a SH3 domain that has been shown to interact with phosphatidylinositol 3 kinase (Prasad *et al,* 1993), an interaction that in turn could allow this lipid kinase to become associated with the T cell receptor–CD3 complex during T cell activation. Thus, $p59^{fyn}$ has the dual function of acting as a kinase as well as mediating molecular associations. The latter role may be especially important, as is suggested for the NCK protein, which consists of one SH2 and three SH3 domains only (Park and Rhee, 1992). The structure of NCK suggests that it acts as an "adaptor" protein binding via its SH2 domain newly tyrosine phosphorylated proteins, which are thus brought into close contact (ie complexed) with proteins binding independently to the SH3 domains. As NCK is itself phosphorylated on tyrosine upon T cell activation, it has the potential of promoting yet further interactions.

## TYROSINE PHOSPHORYLATED PROTEINS

The host of polypeptides phosphorylated on tyrosine in response to T cell activation incorporates a growing number of known proteins, including CD3 $\zeta$ chain, CD5 (Davies *et al,* 1992), CD6 (Wee *et al,* 1993), CD28 (Pages *et al,* 1994) and CD45 (Autero *et al,* 1994) antigens, as well as the PTK ZAP70 (Chan *et al,* 1992), phospholipase C isoforms $\gamma_1$ and $\gamma_2$ (Ettehadieh *et al,* 1992), the proto-oncogene $p95^{vav}$ (Margolis *et al,* 1992) and $\alpha$ tubulin (Ley *et al,* 1994b). Ideally, however, there is a requirement to designate all of the tyrosine phosphorylated polypeptides, including those of low abundance, as well as to describe their respective functions and how these are modulated by phosphorylation/dephosphorylation.

Direct purification and subsequent characterization of the individual polypeptides represents one strategy, although this approach is inevitably qualified by the relatively small amounts of some polypeptides and by the large numbers of tyrosine phosphorylated polypeptides, together with specifically associated (eg via SH2 and SH3 domain mediated interactions) non-phosphorylated polypeptides. Apart from the source of activated T cells, important variables are the choice of detergent employed for cell lysis, the use of phosphatase inhibitors and the choice of the ligand(s) for affinity purification. Although peripheral blood T lymphocytes activated via the T cell receptor complex approximate most closely to the physiological situation of antigen stimulated cells, this choice is ruled out for purification purposes by lack of large number of cells. In our experiments, we have used $5 \times 10^{10}$ batches of cultured T leukaemia Jurkat J6 cells, which had been activated for 90 seconds by cross linking the CD3 antigen with the monoclonal antibody (mAb) UCHT1. With regard to the detergent, by using detergents such as digitonin or BRIJ 96 (Davies *et al,* 1992), it is possible to couple the preservation of macromolecular complexes with effective cell lysis, although it can be difficult to distinguish rigorously between a specific molecular association and ineffective dispersion. We have employed the more dispersive detergent, Nonidet P40, although in this case because of the preservation of an intact cytoskeleton, associated cytoskeleton polypeptides are discarded along with the nuclear fraction. Effective inhibition of tyrosine phosphatases is a prerequisite; a spectrum of inhibitors have been employed, of which sodium vanadate is a most important component. The choice of ligand for affinity purification lies between monoclonal antibodies against phosphotyrosine, such as 4G10 and PY72, and the SH2 domains of the PTKs $p56^{lck}$ and/or $p59^{fyn}$ expressed as fusion proteins.

## SH2 DOMAINS RECOGNIZE AN OVERLAPPING SUBSET OF TYROSINE PHOSPHORYLATED POLYPEPTIDES

A comparison of the specificities of the $p56^{lck}$ and $p59^{fyn}$ SH2 domains with those of phosphotyrosine monoclonal antibodies for the tyrosine phosphorylated polypeptides of activated Jurkat cells is shown in Fig. 1. In particular, the SH2 domains of $p56^{lck}$ and $p59^{fyn}$ precipitated a similar complement of tyrosine phosphorylated polypeptides, which represented a distinct subset of those precipitated by the phosphotyrosine mAb PY72. Specificity of the SH2 domain interaction was proven by demonstrating that a mutant $p56^{lck}$ SH2 domain, in which isoleucine had been replaced by valine, precipitated a much smaller number of polypeptides. Furthermore, when the expressed SH2

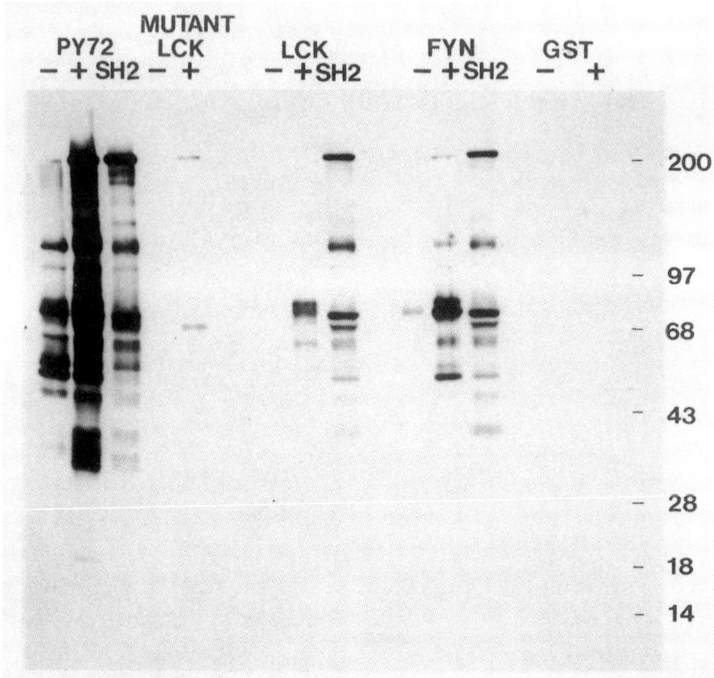


**Fig. 1.** The expressed $p56^{lck}$ and $p59^{fyn}$ SH2 domain-GST fusion proteins precipitate a similar subset of tyrosine phosphorylated proteins. The specificity of binding of the SH2-GST fusion proteins was shown by competitive immunoblotting experiments, in which the pattern of immunoprecipitation of tyrosine phosphorylated proteins by the anti-phosphotyrosine antibody PY72 was altered upon the addition of $p59^{fyn}$ SH2 fusion protein to lysates of activated T cells. The relative intensity was also affected, indicating that the SH2 domains may have a non-specific as well as a specific affinity for tyrosine phosphorylated proteins. The specificity of the SH2 domains for tyrosine phosphorylated proteins was indicated by the lack of binding of the GST protein alone and by a mutation of the $p56^{lck}$ SH2 domain in which isoleucine was replaced by valine. The latter change resulted in a reduced affinity of the domain for tyrosine phosphorylated proteins. Most importantly, the results indicate that the SH2 domains interacted with a subset of the tyrosine phosphorylated proteins, suggesting that they possess a specificity greater than that of the phosphotyrosine antibody. Nonidet P40 lysates from unactivated (−) or CD3 mAb activated (+) $2 \times 10^8$ Jurkat J6 cells were precipitated overnight with a phosphotyrosine antibody (PY72) or with SH2-GST fusion proteins or GST alone. In the case of the SH2 fusion proteins, 25 μl of sonicated bacterial extract was precoupled to 25 μl of glutathione agarose beads, which were then washed three times in phosphate buffered saline, 1% Triton X-100, 100 mmol/l EDTA. The phosphotyrosine mAb PY72 was coupled to protein A Sepharose at 2 mg/ml. The immunoprecipitated proteins were transferred onto polyvinylidene difluoride membrane and immunoblotted with a second phosphotyrosine antibody 4G10. For the precipitate labelled "SH2", 100 μl of sonicated bacterial extract from the $p59^{fyn}$ SH2 expressing bacteria was added to the precipitates of activated J6 cells resulting in a threefold increase relative to the amount of $p59^{fyn}$ SH2 present on the glutathione beads, as determined by protein staining. The same quantity of $p59^{fyn}$ SH2 was added to the PY72 immunoprecipitation. The free SH2 domain resulted in a reduction in the number of proteins immunoprecipitated by PY72

domains were used in competition with the mAb PY72, there was a selective depletion of the bands bound by the monoclonal antibody that were well

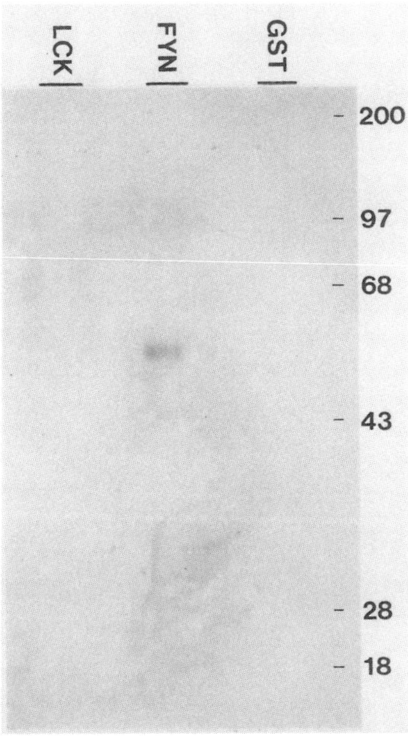


**Fig. 2.** The p56$^{lck}$ and p59$^{fyn}$ SH2 domains possess overlapping but different specifities. Differences in the interactions of the two SH2 domains were revealed by immunoblotting the respective precipitates with a CD5 mAb. In these circumstances, the p59$^{fyn}$, but not the p56$^{lck}$, SH2 domain precipitated the CD5 antigen. Nonidet P40 lysates from CD3 mAb activated (+) 2 x $10^8$ Jurkat J6 cells were precipitated overnight with a phosphotyrosine antibody (4G10), with SH2-GST fusion proteins or GST alone. For the fusion proteins, 25 μl of glutathione agarose beads were added to 100 μl of sonicated bacterial extract during the overnight precipitation; the antibody 4G10 was precoupled to protein A Sepharose at 2 mg/ml. The precipitates were transferred onto PVDF membrane and immunoblotted with a rabbit anti-(CD5) serum

represented in the SH2 precipitate. These results argue strongly that the p56$^{lck}$ or p59$^{fyn}$ SH2 domains represent valuable affinity reagents for the subfractionation of the polypeptides selected by monoclonal antibodies against phosphotyrosine from activated Jurkat cells.

A more detailed comparison of the tyrosine phosphorylated polypeptides precipitated by the p56$^{lck}$ and p59$^{fyn}$ SH2 domains revealed some interesting differences. Thus, as shown in Fig. 2, immunoblotting with a CD5 antiserum indicated that the tyrosine phosphorylated CD5 antigen of activated Jurkat cells (Davies *et al*, 1992) was precipitated by the p59$^{fyn}$ SH2 but not by the p56$^{lck}$ SH2 domain. A similar analysis with a CD7 monoclonal antibody revealed the reverse relationship in preliminary experiments, namely interaction with the p56$^{lck}$ SH2 but not with the p59$^{fyn}$ SH2 domain. In addition, studies by da Silva *et al* (1993) have shown that the p59$^{fyn}$ SH2 domain interacts specifically with a p120/130 polypeptide.

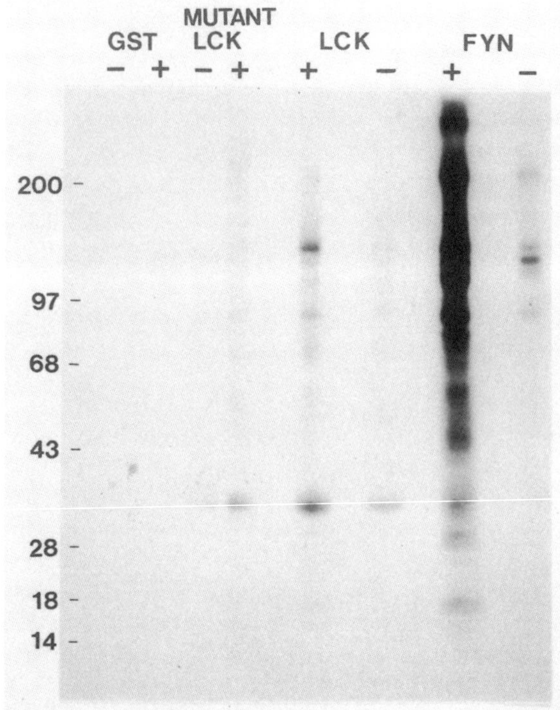


**Fig. 3.** In vitro kinase assays of p56$^{lck}$ and p59$^{fyn}$ SH2 precipitates from activated T cells. The p59$^{fyn}$ SH2 precipitate showed a dramatic increase in associated kinase activity upon T cell activation, and the p56$^{lck}$ SH2 precipitate contained a predominant p35 substrate. This substrate may associate independently of the SH2 domain's ability to bind to tyrosine phosphorylated proteins because the mutant p56$^{lck}$ SH2 domain also bound a p35 polypeptide (Fig. 1). Nonidet P40 lysates from unactivated (−) or CD3 mAb activated (+) 5 x $10^7$ Jurkat J6 cells were precipitated overnight with p56$^{lck}$ and p59$^{fyn}$ SH2-GST fusion proteins in the presence of the tyrosine phosphatase inhibitors 1 mmol/l sodium vanadate and 100 µl phenyl arsine oxide. The precipitations were performed using 50 µl of glutathione agarose beads and 50 µl of sonicated bacterial extract expressing SH2-GST fusion protein or GST alone. The precipitated proteins were assayed for kinase activity in vitro by adding 10 µCi [γ-$^{32}$P]ATP for 15 min. Radioactive bands were revealed by overnight exposure

Another way of analysing the complement of polypeptides precipitated by SH2 domains is by in vitro kinase assays. Figure 3 shows that this approach demonstrated differences in the specificities of p56$^{lck}$ and p59$^{fyn}$ SH2 domains. Thus, the p59$^{fyn}$ SH2 precipitate contained a higher level of kinase activity and gave a different pattern of phosphorylated polypeptides than the p56$^{lck}$ SH2 precipitate, with the principal difference being the presence of a p35 polypeptide in the latter precipitate. As the SH2 domain is devoid of kinase activity, phosphorylation must be due to an associated kinase. Furthermore, since it appears that the kinase activity is principally derived from activated T cells, it follows that either the kinase or its substrates were phosphorylated on tyrosine upon activation.

## FRACTIONATION AND CHARACTERIZATION OF TYROSINE PHOSPHORYLATION POLYPEPTIDES

Affinity chromatography, using phosphotyrosine monoclonal antibodies and/or expressed SH2 domains, represents a powerful selective method for the initial separation of the polypeptides phosphorylated on tyrosine during T lymphocyte activation. Further subfractionation of the selected polypeptides has been achieved by varying the elution conditions in order to differentiate polypeptides binding with different affinities; and by exploiting the differential specificities of the $p56^{lck}$ and $p59^{fyn}$ SH2 domains compared with each other and with monoclonal antibodies. For example, the tyrosine phosphorylated proto-oncogene $p95^{vav}$ was bound by the phosphotyrosine monoclonal antibodies only. In addition, affinity based procedures have been used in combination with conventional methods, such as fine performance liquid chromatography and/or gel filtration. Application of these approaches, either separately or in combination, to batches of about $5 \times 10^{10}$ Jurkat cells stimulated for 90 seconds with the CD3 mAb UCHT1, has provided polypeptides in a form amenable to characterization.

Characterization of the fractionated polypeptides, after further separation by SDS-polyacrylamide gel electrophoresis, has been approached in a variety of ways. In some instances, the application of specific antisera, chosen at random or based on hunches, can provide a robust identification, as in the case of the CD5 antigen (Davies *et al,* 1992). However, procedures that are more guaranteed on providing a positive outcome rely principally upon microsequencing of the eluted bands, either directly from the N-terminus or indirectly by using purified peptides produced by protease digestion. Comparison of the resultant sequences with a sequence database for all known proteins provides either a positive identification or the indication that the polypeptide is not known. The application of this approach to a variety of purified fractions derived from activated Jurkat cells is illustrated in Fig. 4; the corporate results are summarized in Table 1.

Figure 4 compares the polypeptide compositions of various purified fractions, as revealed by protein stains, with the tyrosine phosphorylated band patterns shown by western blotting with the mAb 4G10. Although a number of bands were revealed by both procedures, there were several prominent polypeptides in each fraction that were not coincident with a tyrosine phosphorylated band. For example, fraction number 5 contained a prominent polypeptide of about 100 kDa that was revealed by the protein stain but not by immunoblotting with an antiphosphotyrosine antibody, 4G10. This lack of coincidence could represent a polypeptide impurity contaminating the affinity purified fraction or a non-tyrosine phosphorylated polypeptide that interacts specifically with a tyrosine phosphorylated polypeptide.

As demonstrated in Table 1, microsequence analysis has identified the human homologue of the porcine PTK SYK (Law *et al,* 1994) and an $\alpha$ tubulin (Ley *et al,* 1994b), which are known to be tyrosine phosphorylated on T cell activation. Several apparently non-tyrosine phosphorylated polypeptides were

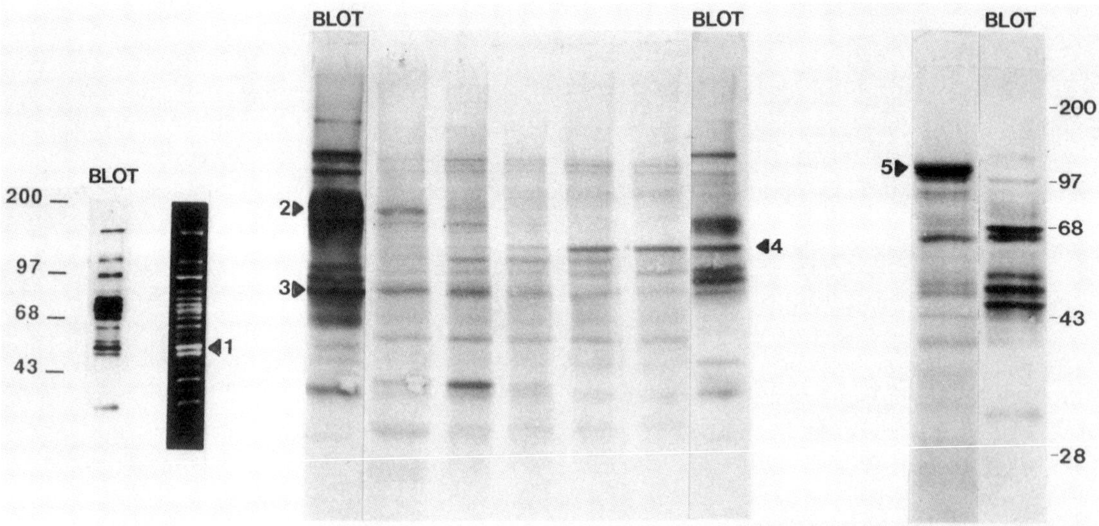


**Fig. 4.** Comparison of polypeptide composition of fractions derived from activated Jurkat T cells by affinity chromatography using the phosphotyrosine mAb 4G10 in combination with fine performance liquid chromatography. Purified fractions were subject to SDS-polyacrylamide gel electrophoresis. Gels were stained using protein dyes, and for some tracks an adjacent lane (blot) was probed for tyrosine phosphorylated polypeptides by western blotting with the mAb 4G10. The bands microsequenced were β tubulin (1), SYK (2), vimentin (3), an unidentified 60 kDa protein (4) and nucleolin (5)

identified, including nucleolin, a known 105 kDa phosphoprotein (Fang and Yeh, 1993); vimentin, a 56 kDa filament protein (Lai *et al,* 1993) that might act as a phosphate "sink" during periods of "excess kinase activity"; and β tubulin, a 50 kDa major component of microtubules. The identification of α tubulin as a target for tyrosine phosphorylation is consistent with the previous demonstra-

**TABLE 1. Characterization by microsequencing of polypeptides purified by affinity chromatography using the phosphotyrosine mAb 4G10[a]**

| Polypeptide | kDa |
|---|---|
| β-tubulin | 50 |
| α-tubulin | 55 |
| Vimentin | 56 |
| p60[b] | 60 |
| SYK | 70 |
| ZAP70 | 70 |
| Nucleolin | 100 |

[a]Polypeptides are listed in order of increasing molecular size, as determined by SDS-polyacrylamide gel electrophoresis (Fig. 4)
[b]An unknown polypeptide of 60 kDa; sequence not represented in the database

tion that receptor tyrosine kinases activate the microtubule associated protein kinase cascade via the SH2/SH3 adaptor proteins, Sos and c-ras (Blenis, 1993).

A method has been described (Pappin *et al,* 1993) for identifying polypeptides by comparing "mass fingerprints" of protease digests determined by mass spectrometry, with a computer generated peptide mass database for all known protein sequences. Application of this procedure to 32 bands eluted from SDS-polyacrylamide gels of affinity purified fractions resulted in positive identification of the polypeptides listed in Table 1. A serine threonine kinase Tpl-2 (tumour progression locus 2; Patriotis *et al,* 1993) is thus identified as a potential phosphorylation intermediate in the T cell activation response pathway. A further four bands gave reasonable mass spectra from protease digests but could not be matched to any of those represented in the database, suggesting that these polypeptides are not presently known; the remaining bands gave insufficient data for analysis.

## CONCLUSION

The identification of the polypeptides that are phosphorylated on tyrosine in response to the initiation of T cell activation by cross linking the T cell receptor–CD3 complex, although desirable, is a daunting task because of the large number of tyrosine phosphorylated polypeptides. The low abundance of some polypeptides and the specific association of some non-phosphorylated polypeptides due to SH2 domain mediated and other specific molecular interactions make the task even harder. Undoubtedly, polypeptide identification will be aided in the future through the application of emerging techniques of characterization, such as those based on mass spectrometric analyses, that are applicable to much smaller amounts of material, as well as to the general increase in the total number of characterized polypeptides due especially to gene cloning. Application of such procedures will inevitably identify previously unknown polypeptides, which thus will also become candidates for gene cloning.

Mere identification of all the polypeptides is, though, of limited value. Identification is solely a step in a longer pathway that has as its ultimate goal the description of the biological activities of the individual polypeptides and how these activities interrelate one to another and are modulated by phosphorylation/dephosphorylation. An especially important criterion will be the designation of those polypeptides that interact specifically to form macromolecular complexes. Such complexes may be transient, may be modulated by phosphorylation and may provide a mechanism for transducing a signal(s) along a pathway(s); in particular, the function(s) of such complexes is most probably a unique property of the complex. Studies of biological function will be promoted through identification of sequence homologies with known functions (eg tyrosine kinase and SH2 domains), through the designation of intracellular location(s), especially if there is an association with a subcellular structure of known function (eg the association of $p59^{fyn}$ with the centrosome;

Ley *et al,* 1994a), and through gene "knockouts". However, it is in the definition of macromolecular complexes that the greatest challenges lie. In this respect, there is a compelling requirement for methodologies that will permit the isolation of further interacting components of a multicomponent complex. Application of such approaches will hopefully lead to the discovery of novel important molecules. With regard to the initiation of T cell activation, the actual initiating molecular event of the tyrosine phosphorylation pathway is still elusive. The possibility that the tyrosine phosphatase activity, which switches on the PTKs $p59^{fyn}$ and ZAP70, is regulated by a specific ligand located on the surface of the antigen presenting cell is especially attractive. In this case, the description of the ligand could provide the clue to the initiating event.

## Acknowledgements

We thank Dr SC Ley and Dr N Osman for their advice and help during the experiments, Dr D Pappin and Iain Goldsmith and their teams at ICRF for their invaluable help in sequencing of peptides and in the synthesis of oligos and Mrs G Paine for help in typing the manuscript.

## References

Anderson D, Koch CA, Grey L, Ellis C, Moran MF and Pawson T (1990) Binding of SH2 domains of phospholipase C gamma 1, GAP, and Src to activated growth factor receptors. *Science* **250** 979–982

Autero M, Saharinen J, Pessa-Morikawa T *et al* (1994) Tyrosine phosphorylation of CD45 phosphotyrosine phosphatase by p50csk kinase creates a binding site for p56lck tyrosine kinase and activates the phosphatase. *Molelcular and Cellular Biology* **14** 1308–1321

Bierer BE, Sleckman BP, Ratnofsky SE and Burakoff SJ (1989) The biologic roles of CD2, CD4, and CD8 in T-cell activation. *Annual Reviews of Immunology* **7** 579–599

Blenis J (1993) Signal transduction via the MAP kinases: proceed at your own risk. *Proceedings of the National Academy of Sciences of the USA* **90** 5889–5892

Boyer C, Ley SC, Davies AA and Crumpton MJ (1993) Comparative analysis of phosphotyrosyl polypeptides in normal and leukemic human T lymphocytes activated via CD3 or CD2. *Molecular Immunology* **30** 903–910

Chan AC, Iwashima M, Turck CW and Weiss A (1992) ZAP-70: a 70 kd protein-tyrosine kinase that associates with the TCR zeta chain. *Cell* **71** 649–662

Clevers H, Alarcon B, Wileman T and Terhorst C (1988) The T cell receptor/CD3 complex: a dynamic protein ensemble. *Annual Reviews of Immunology* **6** 629–662

Collins TL and Burakoff SJ (1993) Tyrosine kinase activity of CD4-associated p56lck may not be required for CD4-dependant T-cell activation. *Proceedings of the National Academy of Sciences of the USA* **90** 11885–11889

da Silva AJ, Janssen O and Rudd CE (1993) T cell receptor zeta/CD3-p59fyn(T)-associated p120/130 binds to the SH2 domain of p59fyn(T). *Journal of Experimental Medicine* **178** 2107–2113

Davies AA, Ley SC and Crumpton MJ (1992) CD5 is phosphorylated on tyrosine after stimulation of the T-cell antigen receptor complex. *Proceedings of the National Academy of Sciences of the USA* **89** 6368–6372

Downward J, Graves JD and Cantrell D (1992) The regulation and function of p21ras in T cells. *Immunology Today* **13** 89–92

Eck MJ, Atwell SK, Shoelson SE and Harrison SC (1994) Structure of the regulatory domains of the src-family tyrosine kinase lck. *Nature* **368** 764–769

Ettehadieh E, Sanghera JS, Pelech SL *et al* (1992) Tyrosyl phosphorylation and activation of MAP kinases by p56lck. *Science* **255** 853–855

Iwashima M, Irving BA, van Oers NS, Chan AC and Weiss A (1994) Sequential interactions of the TCR with two distinct cytoplasmic tyrosine kinases. *Science* **263** 1136–1139

Lai YK, Lee WC and Chen KD (1993) Vimentin serves as a phosphate sink during the apparent activation of protein kinases by okadaic acid in mammalian cells. *Journal of Cellular Biochemistry* **53** 161–168

Law CL, Sidorenko SP, Chandran KA *et al* (1994) Molecular cloning of human Syk: a B cell protein-tyrosine kinase associated with the surface immunoglobulin M-B cell receptor complex. *Journal of Biological Chemistry* **269** 12310–12319

Lee S-K, Su B, Maher SE and Bothwell ALM (1994) Ly-6A is required for T cell receptor expression and protein tyrosine kinase fyn activity. *EMBO Journal* **13** 2167–2176

Ley SC, Davies AA, Druker B and Crumpton MJ (1991) The T cell receptor/CD3 complex and CD2 stimulate the tyrosine phosphorylation of indistinguishable patterns of polypeptides in the human T leukemic cell line Jurkat. *European Journal of Immunology* **21** 2203–2209

Ley SC, Marsh M, Bebbington CR, Proudfoot K and Jordan P (1994a) Distinct intracellular-localization of lck and fyn protein-tyrosine kinases in human T-lymphocytes. *Journal of Cell Biology* **125** 639–649

Ley SC, Verbi W, Pappin DJC, Druker B, Davies AA and Crumpton MJ (1994b) Tyrosine phosphorylation of alpha-tubulin in human T-lymphocytes. *European Journal of Immunology* **24** 99–106

Luo KX and Sefton BM (1990) Cross-linking of T-cell surface molecules CD4 and CD8 stimulates phosphorylation of the lck tyrosine protein kinase at the autophosphorylation site. *Molecular and Cellular Biology* **10** 5305–5313

McFarland ED, Hurley TR, Pingel JT, Sefton BM, Shaw A and Thomas ML (1993) Correlation between Src family member regulation by the protein-tyrosine-phosphatase CD45 and transmembrane signalling through the T-cell receptor. *Proceedings of the National Academy of Sciences of the USA* **90** 1402–1406

Marengere LEM, Songyang Z, Gish GD *et al* (1994) SH2 domain specificity and activity modified by a single residue. *Nature* **369** 502–505

Margolis B, Hu P, Katzav S *et al* (1992) Tyrosine phosphorylation of *vav* proto-oncogene product containing SH2 domain and transcription factor motifs. *Nature* **356** 71–74

Pages F, Raguencau M, Rotlapel R *et al* (1994) Binding of phosphatidyl-inositol-3-OH kinase to CD28 is required for T-cell signalling. *Nature* **369** 327–329

Pappin DJC, Hojrup P and Bleasby AJ (1993) Rapid identification of proteins by peptide-mass fingerprinting. *Current Biology* **3** 327–332

Park D and Rhee SG (1992) Phosphorylation of Nck in response to a variety of receptors, phorbol myristate acetate and cyclic AMP. *Molecular and Cellular Biology* **12** 5816–5823

Patriotis C, Makris A, Bear SE and Tsichlis PN (1993) Tumour progression locus 2 (Tpl-2) encodes a protein kinase involved in the progression of rodent T-cell lymphomas and in T-cell activation. *Proceedings of the National Academy of Sciences of the USA* **90** 2251–2255

Prasad KV, Janssen O, Kapeller R, Raab M, Cantley LC and Rudd CE (1993) Src-homology 3 domain of protein kinase p59fyn mediates binding to phosphatidylinositol 3-kinase in T cells. *Proceedings of the National Academy of Sciences of the USA* **90** 7366–7370

Samelson LE and Klausner RD (1993) Tyrosine kinases and tyrosine-based activation motifs: current research on activation via the T cell antigen receptor. *Journal of Biological Chemistry* **267** 24913–24916

Sieh M, Bolen JB and Weiss A (1993) CD45 specifically modulates binding of Lck to a phosphopeptide encompassing the negative regulatory tyrosine of Lck. *EMBO Journal* **12** 315–321

Songyang Z, Shoelson SE, Chaudhuri M *et al* (1993) SH2 domains recognize specific phosphopeptide sequences. *Cell* **72** 767–778

Spertini F, Stohl W, Ramesh N, Moody C and Geha RS (1991) Induction of human T cell proliferation by a monoclonal antibody to CD5. *Journal of Immunology* **146** 47–52

Veillette A and Davidson D (1993) Src-related protein tyrosine kinases and T-cell receptor signalling. *Trends in Genetics* **8** 61–66

Veillette A, Bolen JB and Brookman MA (1989) Induction of human T cell proliferation by a monoclonal antibody to CD5. *Journal of Immunology* **146** 47–52

Waksman G, Kominos D, Robertson SC *et al* (1992) Crystal structure of the phosphotyrosine recognition domain SH2 of v-src complexed with tyrosine-phosphorylated peptides. *Nature* **358** 646–653

Wee SF, Schieven GL, Kurihara JM *et al* (1993) Tyrosine phosphorylation of CD6 by stimulation of CD3: augmentation by the CD4 and CD2 coreceptors. *Journal of Experimental Medicine* **177** 219–223

Weiss A (1993) T cell antigen receptor signal transduction: a tale of tails and cytoplasmic protein-tyrosine kinases. *Cell* **73** 209–212

Weiss A, Koretzky G, Schatzman RC and Kadlecek T (1991) Functional activation of the T-cell antigen receptor induces tyrosine phosphorylation of phospholipase C-gamma 1. *Proceedings of the National Academy of Sciences of the USA* **88** 5484–5488

The authors are responsible for the accuracy of the references.

# Biographical Notes

**Sir Walter Bodmer,** director-general of the Imperial Cancer Research Fund, read mathemetatics at Cambridge University and went on to obtain a PhD in population genetics. He spent 9 years at Stanford University, California, working with Joshua Lederberg, before taking up an appointment as professor of genetics at Oxford University in 1970. In 1979 he became director of research at the Imperial Cancer Research Fund and was appointed director-general in 1991. He is also chairman of the Committee on the Public Understanding of Science and president of the International Human Genome Organization. His research interests centre on the expression of HLA determinants in cancer and the genetics and biology of the epithelial cells in the colon, from which the majority of colorectal adenocarcinomas are derived.

**Doreen Cantrell** graduated BSc from the University of Wales in 1979 and obtained her PhD from Nottingham University in 1982. In 1984 she joined ICRF as a postdoctoral fellow with Dr MJ Crumpton and is now a senior scientist at ICRF, responsible for the lymphocyte activation laboratory. Her research interest is the regulation of the activation and proliferation of T lymphocytes.

**Michael Crumpton** is chief operating officer at Imperial Cancer Research Fund Technology Limited, London. He graduated in chemistry at the then University College, Southampton, in 1950 and obtained his PhD at the Lister Institute of Preventive Medicine, London, in 1953. He joined RR Porter at the Wright-Fleming Institute and in 1966 went to the National Institute for Medical Research, eventually becoming head of the division of biochemistry. He moved to the ICRF in 1979 as deputy director of research and in the same year was elected a Fellow of the Royal Society. From 1991 to 1993 he was director of research and was made Commander of the British Empire in 1992 for services to science.

**Frances Gotch,** PhD, trained in immunology at the National Institute for Medical Research with Professor John Humphreys. Since 1979 she has worked with Professor Andrew McMichael in Oxford on virus specific MHC restricted cytotoxic T cell responses in man and in animal models. She is a research scientist in the molecular immunology group in the Institute of Molecular Medicine. Her main interest currently is the role of cytotoxic T lymphocytes in human immunodeficiency virus infection.

**Howard M Grey** graduated MD from New York University. After working as an assistant professor at Rockefeller University and later as an associate member in the department of experimental pathology at Scripps Clinic and Research Foundation in La Jolla, California, he moved to the National Jewish Hospital and Research Center in Denver, Colorado, in 1970. From 1978 to 1988 he was head of the division of basic immunology at the National Jewish Center for Immunology and Respiratory Medicine (formerly the National Jewish Hospital and Research Center) in Denver. He was an associate professor of pathology from 1970 to 1975 and a professor of pathology from 1976 to 1988 at the University of Colorado Medical Center in Denver. He was founder of Cytel and since 1988 has been vice-president of research and development.

**David Jackson** gained his DPhil at Oxford University, studying the heterogeneity of CD45 antigen under the supervision of Dr AN Barclay. He did postdoctoral research in plant virology at Imperial College, London, then joined ICRF as a senior scientific officer under Dr P Goodfellow, before returning to immunology by joining Dr MJ Crumpton's laboratory.

**W Martin Kast** received his PhD from the University of Amsterdam in 1987. He joined the division of immunology at the Netherlands Cancer Institute in Amsterdam, where he held the position of staff member until 1990. Presently he is head of the tumour immunology section of the department of immunohaematology and blood bank, Academic Hospital, University of Leiden, and a senior fellow of the Royal Academy of Arts and Sciences.

**Paul Klennerman** graduated in medicine from Oxford University in 1988. He is currently working as a Wellcome Trust training fellow with Dr Rodney Phillips and Professor Andrew McMichael on the cytotoxic T cell response to human immunodeficiency virus.

**Ralph T Kubo** received his PhD from the University of Hawaii in 1970 and was an assistant professor there until 1971. From 1971 to 1980 he worked in the division of basic immunology, department of medicine, at the National Jewish Center for Immunology and Respiratory Medicine in Denver, Colarado. He was also an associate professor in the department of medicine from 1980 to 1989, and a professor in the department of microbiology and immunology from 1989 to 1991, at the University of Colorado Health Sciences Center in Denver. In 1991 he joined Cytel as a principal scientist in the department of immunology.

**Andrew Lazarovitz** gained his MD at McMaster University in 1978 and went on to specialize in nephrology. He is an associate professor of medicine, microbiology and immunology and director of renal transplantation at the University of Western Ontario. He is also active in the field of T cell research, CD7 and CD45 antigens being among his main interests.

**Andrew McMichael** graduated in medicine from the University of Cambridge in 1968. He trained in immunology at the National Institute for Medical Research with Dr AR Williamson and Dr BA Askonas, obtaining his PhD in 1974. After two years with Dr Hugh McDevitt at Stanford University, he took up an appointment in Oxford in 1977. Since then, he has developed an interest in the role of cytotoxic T lymphocytes in human immune responses, with particular reference to the function of HLA class I antigens. He was appointed to a Medical Research Council clinical research professorship in 1982.

**Stefan C Meuer,** MD, is head of the division of applied immunology at the German Cancer Research Centre and holds an appointment as professor of applied immunology in the medical faculty at the University of Heidelberg. His research interests include molecular and clinical aspects of T lymphocyte activation, with the goal of developing new diagnostic tools as well as novel approaches to clinical immune intervention.

**Paul Moss** graduated in medicine from Cambridge University and completed his clinical training at Oxford. His research interest is the human T cell receptor and in particular T cell recognition in viral infections. He combines this with clinical training in haematology.

**Stanley G Nathenson** is professor of cell biology and professor of microbiology and immunology at Albert Einstein College of Medicine, New York, having joined the school in 1965. He graduated from the Washington University School of Medicine in 1959, and then worked as a fellow of the Helen Hay Whitney Foundation. In 1988 he was elected to the National Academy of Sciences. His work has been concerned with investigating the functional properties of the products of the major histocompatibility class I complex at a structural level.

**Michael J Owen** graduated in biochemistry from Oxford University, took his PhD at Cambridge University and was a postdoctoral fellow at the National Institute for Medical Research, London, and at Massachusetts Institute of Technology. He joined ICRF in 1979 and is now head of the laboratory of lymphocyte molecular biology. His research interest is molecular immunology and is focused on the T cell receptor and the molecular basis of thymocyte differentiation.

**Manuel Izquierdo Pastor** obtained his PhD at the University of Madrid in 1990 and joined ICRF as a postdoctoral research fellow the same year. In 1993 he returned to Spain to take up a postdoctoral position in the University of Granada. His research interest is the control of T cell growth and apoptosis, with a particular focus on the cellular biochemistry of these events.

**Roger M Perlmutter** received MD and PhD degrees from Washington University, St Louis, where he studied the molecular heterogeneity of anti-carbohydrate antibodies under Joseph M Davie. After clinical training in internal medicine at Massachusetts General Hospital and the University of California, San Francisco, he spent three years at the California Institute of Technology, working with Leroy E Hood. He then joined the University of Washington School of Medicine, where he is currently an investigator at the Howard Hughes Medical Institute, professor and chairman of the department of immunology and professor of medicine and biochemistry.

**Sarah Rowland-Jones** graduated in medicine in 1983 after studies in the Universities of Cambridge and Oxford and then spent a period of further training in general medicine and infectious diseases in London, Sheffield and Oxford. Since 1989 she has been with the molecular immunology group in Oxford, studying the role of HIV specific cytotoxic T lymphocytes in the natural history of infection with the human immunodeficiency virus.

**Jörg Ruppert** graduated in immunology from the University of Göttingen, Germany, in 1991, with a fellowship from the Boehringer Ingelheim Foundation. In 1990 he was a visiting scientist at the University of Southern California Medical School in Los Angeles, with W John Martin's group. In 1991 he joined Cytel as a research scientist in the department of immunology, working with Howard Grey and Alessandro Sette.

**James C Sacchettini** received his PhD in molecular biology from Washington University, St Louis, in 1987. He spent two further years there, first as a postdoctoral fellow, then as research assistant professsor in the department of biochemistry and molecular biophysics. Since 1990 he has been assistant professor in the department of biochemistry at Albert Einstein College of Medicine, New York. His work entails X ray crystallographic studies of a variety of biological molecules, including those involved in cellular immunity, in order to elucidate their structure and mode of action.

**Yvonne Samstag,** MD, is a group leader in the division of applied immunology at the German Cancer Research Centre. Her research interests relate to mechanisms of signal transduction in human T cells, with special emphasis on accessory receptor dependent signalling reactions.

**Burkhart Schraven,** MD, is a group leader in the division of applied immunology at the German Cancer Research Centre. His major area of research is the molecular analysis of accessory receptor complexes in human T cells and their associated signalling proteins.

**Alessandro Sette** received his PhD from the University of Rome in 1984. After working as a postdoctoral fellow with Luciano Adorini in Rome, in 1986 he joined Howard Grey's laboratory at the National Jewish Center for Immunology and Respiratory Medicine in Denver, Colorado. He joined Cytel in 1988 as a staff scientist and since 1993 has been director of immunochemistry. In addition, since 1988 he has been an adjunct member of the department of immunology at the Research Institute of Scripps Clinic in La Jolla, California.

**John Sidney** joined the department of immunochemistry at Cytel in 1988. He is a senior research associate and a specialist in the computer analysis of peptide binding data.

**Winston Verbi** is a fellow of the Institute of Science and Technology, and his thesis on anti-lymphocyte antibodies was to set a basis for his long and productive career in immunology. After coming to England from Kenya in 1967, he worked as a chief technician/scientific officer for Professors Roitt, Greaves and Mitchison before working for Dr MJ Crumpton at the ICRF. He has now retired from active science and is living in Spain.

**Antonella Vitiello** received her PhD from the University of Pavia in 1972 and was an assistant professor in the clinical immunology group, department of paediatrics, until 1985. She worked in Dr Linda Sherman's laboratory at Scripps Clinic and Research Foundation, La Jolla, California, until 1989, when she joined the department of immunology at Cytel as a staff scientist. Since 1993 she has been a group leader at Cytel.

**Melissa Woodrow,** BSc, is a graduate of the University of Rochester, New York. She joined ICRF in 1990 as a PhD student.

**Aideen C M Young** graduated in physical chemistry from Trinity College, Dublin. She then moved to the United States and received her PhD from New York University. Since January 1992 she has been a postdoctoral fellow working as a crystallographer in the laboratories of Dr J Sacchettini and Dr S Nathenson at the Albert Einstein College of Medicine in New York. In January 1993 she was awarded a postdoctoral fellowship by the Irvington Institute for Medical Research. Her research interest is the structure of murine class I MHC molecules.

**Weiguo Zhang** is studying for a PhD in cell biology at Albert Einstein College of Medicine, New York. He received his BS in genetics from Wuhan University and MS in biochemistry from Fudan University, China. His research interests are the overexpression, in vitro reconstitution and crystal structures of murine class I H-2$K^b$ and $D^b$ molecules.

# Index

# LIST OF PREVIOUS ISSUES

## VOLUME 1 1982

**No. 1: Inheritance of Susceptibility to Cancer in Man**
Guest Editor: W F Bodmer

**No. 2: Maturation and Differentiation in Leukaemias**
Guest Editor: M F Greaves

**No. 3: Experimental Approaches to Drug Targeting**
Guest Editors: A J S Davies and M J Crumpton

**No. 4: Cancers Induced by Therapy**
Guest Editor: I Penn

## VOLUME 2 1983

**No. 1: Embryonic & Germ Cell Tumours in Man and Animals**
Guest Editor: R L Gardner

**No. 2: Retinoids and Cancer**
Guest Editor: M B Sporn

**No. 3: Precancer**
Guest Editor: J J DeCosse

**No. 4: Tumour Promotion and Human Cancer**
Guest Editors: T J Slaga and R Montesano

## VOLUME 3 1984

**No. 1: Viruses in Human and Animal Cancers**
Guest Editors: J Wyke and R Weiss

**No. 2: Gene Regulation in the Expression of Malignancy**
Guest Editor: L Sachs

**No. 3: Consistent Chromosomal Aberrations and Oncogenes in Human Tumours**
Guest Editor: J D Rowley

**No. 4: Clinical Management of Solid Tumours in Childhood**
Guest Editor: T J McElwain

## VOLUME 4 1985

**No. 1: Tumour Antigens in Experimental and Human Systems**
Guest Editor: L W Law

**No. 2: Recent Advances in the Treatment and Research in Lymphoma and Hodgkin's Disease**
Guest Editor: R Hoppe

**No. 3: Carcinogenesis and DNA Repair**
Guest Editor: T Lindahl

**No. 4: Growth Factors and Malignancy**
Guest Editors: A B Roberts and M B Sporn

## VOLUME 5 1986

**No. 1: Drug Resistance**
Guest Editors: G Stark and H Calvert

**No. 2: Biochemical Mechanisms of Oncogene Activity: Proteins Encoded by Oncogenes**
Guest Editors: H E Varmus and J M Bishop

**No. 3: Hormones and Cancer: 90 Years after Beatson**
Guest Editor: R D Bulbrook

**No. 4: Experimental, Epidemiological and Clinical Aspects of Liver Carcinogenesis**
Guest Editor: E Farber

## VOLUME 6 1987

**No. 1: Naturally Occurring Tumours in Animals as a Model for Human Disease**
Guest Editors: D Onions and W Jarrett

**No. 2: New Approaches to Tumour Localization**
Guest Editor: K Britton

**No. 3: Psychological Aspects of Cancer**
Guest Editor: S Greer

**No. 4: Diet and Cancer**
Guest Editors: C Campbell and L Kinlen

## VOLUME 7 1988

**No. 1: Pain and Cancer**
Guest Editor: G W Hanks

**No. 2: Somatic Cell Genetics and Cancer**
Guest Editor: L M Franks

**No. 3: Prospects for Primary and Secondary Prevention of Cervix Cancer**
Guest Editors: G Knox and C Woodman

**No. 4: Tumour Progression and Metastasis**
Guest Editor: I Hart

## VOLUME 8 1989

**No. 1: Colorectal Cancer**
Guest Editor: J Northover

**No. 2: Nitrate, Nitrite and Nitroso Compounds in Human Cancer**
Guest Editors: D Forman and D E G Shuker

**No. 3: A Critical Assessment of Cancer Chemotherapy**
Guest Editor: A H Calvert

**No. 4: Biological Response Modifiers**
Guest Editors: F R Balkwill and W Fiers

## VOLUME 9 1990

**No. 1: Haemopoietic Growth Factors: Their Role in the Treatment of Cancer**
Guest Editor: M Dexter

**No. 2: Germ Cell Tumours of the Testis: A Clinico-Pathological Perspective**
Guest Editors: P Andrews and T Oliver

**No. 3: Genetics and Cancer— Part I**
Guest Editors: W Cavenee, B Ponder and E Solomon

**No. 4: Genetics and Cancer— Part II**
Guest Editors: W Cavenee, B Ponder and E Solomon

## VOLUME 10 1991

**Cancer, HIV and AIDS**
Guest Editors: V Beral, H W Jaffe and R A Weiss

## VOLUME 11 1991

**Prostate Cancer: Cell and Molecular Mechanisms in Diagnosis and Treatment**
Guest Editor: J T Isaacs

**VOLUME 12 1992**

**Tumour Suppressor Genes, the Cell Cycle and Cancer**
Guest Editor: A J Levine

**VOLUME 13 1992**

**A New Look at Tumour Immunology**
Guest Editors: A J McMichael and W F Bodmer

**VOLUME 14 1992**

**Growth Regulation by Nuclear Hormone Receptors**
Guest Editor: M G Parker

**VOLUME 15 1992**

**Oncogenes in the Development of Leukaemia**
Guest Editor: O N Witte

**VOLUME 16 1993**

**The Molecular Pathology of Cancer**
Guest Editors: N R Lemoine and N A Wright

**VOLUME 17 1993**

**Pharmacokinetics and Cancer Chemotherapy**
Guest Editors: P Workman and M A Graham

**VOLUME 18 1993**

**Breast Cancer**
Guest Editors: I S Fentiman and J Taylor-Papadimitriou

**VOLUME 19/20 1994**

**Trends in Cancer Incidence and Mortality**
Guest Editors: R Doll, J F Fraumeni Jr and C S Muir

**VOLUME 21 1994**

**Palliative Medicine: Problem Areas in Pain and Symptom Management**
Guest Editor: G W Hanks